Competencies

for

Staff Educators

TOOLS TO EVALUATE AND ENHANCE NURSING PROFESSIONAL DEVELOPMENT

Barbara A. Brunt, MA, MN, RN,BC

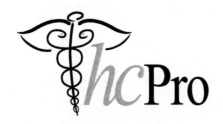

Competencies for Staff Educators: Tools to Evaluate and Enhance Nursing Professional Development
is published by HCPro, Inc.

HCPro, Inc., provides information resources for the healthcare industry. HCPro, Inc. is not affiliated in any way with The Joint Commission, which owns the JCAHO and Joint Commission trademarks.

MAGNET™, MAGNET RECOGNITION PROGRAM®, and ANCC MAGNET RECOGNITION® are trademarks of the American Nurses Credentialing Center (ANCC). The products and services of HCPro, Inc. and The Greeley Company are neither sponsored nor endorsed by the ANCC.

Barbara A. Brunt, MA, MN, RN,BC, Author
Julia Aucoin, DNS, RN, BC, Contributing Author
Rebecca Hendren, Managing Editor
Emily Sheahan, Group Publisher
Shane Katz, Cover Designer
Jackie Diehl Singer, Graphic Artist
Jean St. Pierre, Director of Operations
Darren Kelly, Production Coordinator
Genevieve d'Entremont, Copyeditor
Sada Preisch, Proofreader

Advice given is general. Readers should consult professional counsel for specific legal, ethical, or clinical questions. Arrangements can be made for quantity discounts. For more information, contact

HCPro, Inc.
P.O. Box 1168
Marblehead, MA 01945
Telephone: 800/650-6787 or 781/639-1872
Fax: 781/639-2982
E-mail: *customerservice@hcpro.com*

Visit HCPro, Inc., at its World Wide Web sites: *www.hcpro.com* and *www.hcmarketplace.com*

Rev. 09/2007
21054

DEDICATION

This book is dedicated to three individuals who have passed away, but who had a tremendous impact on my life.

First I want to thank Doris Gosnell, my mentor, colleague, and friend. She decided to take a chance by hiring a nurse with an associate's degree in nursing and a bachelor's degree in education. When I first started my staff development career in 1978, I worked with nursing assistants and other non-professional staff. Through Doris' guidance and mentoring, I assumed more and more responsibility in that department, becoming a coordinator, and then ultimately the director of the department when she retired. She supported me as I went through my master's program in community health education, but always told me I needed to get a master's degree in nursing. I am sorry that she did not live to see me achieve that goal.

Next, I want to acknowledge my late husband, John G. Brunt. In our 34 years of marriage, he always supported my professional nursing endeavors, even though it took away from our time together. He was there as I completed the pilot and first four phases of the research study. I miss his smile, his sense of adventure, and his outgoing disposition.

Finally, I want to acknowledge my father, Raymond G. Johnson. As I worked for him at Johnson's Furniture throughout my junior high and high school years, I developed my work ethic and values, as well as my organizational and communication skills, which have served me well in my career path. He and Mom helped support me financially as I went through college and provided an ongoing source of encouragement throughout my life.

Contents

Competencies for Staff Educators: Tools to Evaluate and Enhance Nursing Professional Development

Contents

LIST OF FIGURES AND EXHIBITS

Barbara A. Brunt, MA, MN, RN,BC

Barbara A. Brunt, MA, MN, RN,BC, is Director of Nursing Education and Staff Development for Summa Health System Hospitals in Akron, OH. She has held a variety of staff development positions, including educator, coordinator, and director, for the past 28 years. Brunt has presented on a variety of topics both locally and nationally, and has published numerous articles and chapters in books. She served as section editor for the first and second editions of *The Core Curriculum for Staff Development*, published by NNSDO, and was part of the task force that revised the *Scope and Standards of Practice for Nursing Professional Development*, published by ANA. She is a coauthor of *Competency Management System: Toolkit for Validation and Assessment*, published by HCPro.

Brunt holds a master's degree in community health education from Kent State University and a master's in nursing from the University of Dundee in Scotland. Her research has focused on competencies. Brunt maintains certification in nursing professional development, as well as medical-surgical nursing. She has been active in numerous professional associations and has received awards for excellence in writing, nursing research, leadership, and staff development. Brunt is serving a term as President-Elect of NNSDO through July of 2007, when she will begin a two-year term as President of that organization.

Contributing author: Julia Aucoin, DNS, RN-BC, CNE

Dr. Julia Aucoin is certified in Nursing Professional Development and Academic Education and has worked on the certification teams with associated competencies for both specialty practices. She has served as a professor in nursing education and as the CE Consultant for the North Carolina Nurses Association, and has held positions as Director of Education in several hospitals. Dr. Aucoin is a frequent presenter at the National Nurses Staff Development Organization (NNSDO) and National League for Nursing's Annual Conventions as well as published on nursing education topics. She is coeditor of *Conversations in Nursing Professional Development*, published by NNSDO.

ACKNOWLEDGMENTS

This book was made possible through the support and assistance of many individuals, and although I cannot recognize everyone who assisted with this endeavor, there are some special people I would like to acknowledge.

First and foremost, I would like to thank the staff development personnel throughout the United States who participated in the research studies that led to the development of the competency assessment tool. I asked for feedback and suggestions on the competencies and performance criteria and received a wealth of information from the respondents. This helped me refine and clarify the competencies and performance expectations.

Julia Aucoin is a dear friend and colleague. She provided support, assistance, and encouragement throughout the entire process. In addition to suggesting I validate the results with academic educators, she helped gather data from a pilot group to gain additional feedback on how the performance criteria fit into Benner's novice-to-expert continuum. She provided specific feedback as I was working on my dissertation, and assisted me as I was trying to find a publisher for my work.

Dr. Liz Rogerson from the University of Dundee in Scotland helped me enhance my critical thinking skills and become a more reflective practitioner. As my dissertation advisor, she provided ongoing feedback in all the stages of this project to help make sense of all the data I had collected.

I would like to thank Summa Health System and particularly Jane Soposky and Cathy Koppelman for their ongoing support of my professional endeavors. Summa Health System Foundation and the Department of Patient Care Services provided financial support for the pilot study through the Clinical Ladder program. The Nursing Research Division also provided data analysis assistance throughout all the phases of the research. In addition, I would like to recognize the financial assistance of the National Nursing Staff Development Organization for research grants for four of the phases of the study, the Delta Omega Chapter of Sigma Theta Tau for partial support of one phase of the study, and the Ohio Nurses Foundation for financial support for one phase of the study.

Last, but certainly not least, I want to acknowledge my daughters, Rhonda Beasley and Becky Brunt, as well as my mother, Betty Johnson. They are an important part of my life and who I am, and I am very lucky to have such wonderful family members who always are there to support and listen to me.

Although the focus on competence in nursing practice is a worldwide phenomenon and there is a lot of literature on educational methods to achieve competence, there is limited literature on nursing professional development (NPD) competencies or effective methods to measure the achievement of competencies by staff development specialists.

This book, which will add to the body of evidence-based staff development literature, is appropriate for staff development or patient educators in any setting. Since many of the educational competencies are similar regardless of practice setting, this may also be helpful as a resource for educators in other settings, such as academia or consultants.

Individuals can take the competencies in this book and immediately incorporate them into their practice. The book focuses on how to use this information in a variety of ways, such as creating an orientation for a new staff development specialist, completing a self-assessment, creating criterion-based job descriptions, or incorporating them as part of a performance development plan. This will provide a consistent, objective, validated tool to assist NPD educators in measuring their competence. With today's emphasis on cost-containment and accountability, it is critical that educators demonstrate their competence.

This book will provide specific performance criteria to evaluate a wide range of professional NPD educator competencies. The author consolidated information from a series of research studies designed to identify and validate specific criteria that determine whether staff development or other educators were meeting various competencies, and also put in a framework to make it easier to use.

The book is divided into three sections. The first section provides an overview of the competency movement and describes how the educational competencies and performance criteria in this book were developed. It describes the framework for the competencies and outlines methods that can be used to validate competence.

The second section provides examples of how the competencies can be used and applied in the practice setting in a variety of roles. Specific areas include self-assessment, criterion-based position descriptions, orientation, performance appraisals, professional portfolios, and cultural competence.

The third section explores other potential uses of the competencies, as well as future trends. The self-assessment tool is included on the accompanying CD-ROM, so readers can easily modify it to meet their individual needs.

SECTION I

Competency assessment and validation

This section provides an overview of the competency movement and describes how the educational competencies and corresponding performance criteria in this book were developed. It describes the framework for the competencies and outlines methods that can be used to validate competence.

Overview of the competency movement

Learning objective

After reading this chapter, the participant should be able to
- discuss key components of competence and competency-based education

Key concepts

Before beginning a discussion of nursing professional development educator competencies, it is important to first discuss the key concepts and definitions. Most of these concepts have been defined by the American Nurses Association (ANA) in their *Scope and Standards of Practice for Nursing Professional Development*.

Competence: A person's capacity to perform his or her job function.

Competency statement: A statement that describes a general or broad area of behavior/performance that is requisite for being competent in a particular role and work setting.

Continuing competence: Ongoing professional nursing competence according to level of expertise, responsibility, and domains of practice, and as evidenced by behavior based on beliefs, attitudes, and knowledge matched to and in the context of a set of expected outcomes as defined by nursing scope of policy, code of ethics, standards, guidelines, and benchmarks that ensure safe performance of professional activities.

Continuing education: Systematic professional learning experiences designed to augment the knowledge, skills, and attitudes of nurses and therefore enrich the nurses' contribution to quality healthcare and their pursuit of professional career goals.

Nursing professional development: The lifelong process of active participation by nurses in learning activities that assist in developing and maintaining their continuing competence, enhance their professional practice, and support achievement of their career goals.

Nursing professional development educator: A registered nurse whose practice is in nursing education and who facilitates lifelong learning in a variety of healthcare, educational, and academic settings.

Performance criteria: Statements that define the critical or essential behaviors that represent a particular competency. These outcomes require integration of learning and application of that learning.

Staff development: The systematic process of assessment, development, and evaluation that enhances the performance or professional development of healthcare providers and their continuing competence, according to the National Nursing Staff Development Organization (NNSDO).

Why is competence important?

Continuing competence is an issue that affects nurses in all practice settings. Society demands that nurses demonstrate their competence, and increased pressure from multiple healthcare regulatory agencies and the public necessitates comprehensive evaluation of staff competency. In addition, the emphasis on evidence-based practice has created increased scrutiny of clinicians and their preparation.

The issue of continued competence will remain a challenge to the health profession for many years. With the never-ending changes in science and technology, the healthcare environment, patient expectations, and regulations, health professionals need to attain and maintain competence throughout their careers. However, definitions of competence and strategies to document competence vary, and there is little evidence to support specific, successful methods for validating competence.

What is competence in nursing?

The focus on competence in nursing is a worldwide phenomenon. Dickenson-Hazard outlined several competence-related themes from a series of global conferences sponsored by the Sigma Theta Tau International Honor Society of Nursing (Dickenson-Hazard 2004). Themes included

- instituting core competencies and standards for professional nursing practice
- developing nurses' competency to assess and use technology
- developing nurses' competency to effectively apply health information
- promoting lifelong learning systems for nurses
- creating evidence-based nursing models
- developing innovative strategies to educate patients, communities, and nurses

Most writers agree that competency is about what someone can do. Competency involves both the ability to perform in a given context and the capacity to transfer knowledge and skills to new tasks and situations. Performance criteria can be used to outline the steps that must be taken to achieve competency.

The role of nursing professional development educators

One of the responsibilities of nursing professional development (NPD) educators is to assess the competencies of nursing staff members. NPD educators play an important role in promoting life-long learning for nurses and documenting the competence of nursing staff members. These educators build on the education and experiential bases of nurses throughout their professional careers, working toward the ultimate goal of ensuring quality healthcare for the public.

Competency-based education

Competency-based education (CBE) is one approach that NPD educators use to assess and validate competence. CBE reflects a pragmatic concern that nurses are able to *do* a task, rather than simply *know* how to do a task. Competency models began to evolve during the 1960s as an approach to education, and today CBE models constitute a widely applied approach to validating competence. With CBE, learning is self-directed, which allows educators to act as facilitators to promote learners' goals. The CBE approach is compatible with adult developmental needs.

Common characteristics of CBE include a learner-centered philosophy, real-life orientation, flexibility, clearly articulated standards, a focus on outcomes, and criterion-reference evaluation methods. CBE emphasizes outcomes in terms of what individuals must know and be able to do, and allows flexible pathways for achieving those outcomes. A comparison of CBE and traditional education is provided in Figure 1.1.

FIGURE 1.1 **Comparison of competency-based education (CBE) and traditional education**

Characteristic	CBE programs (Learner-centered)	Traditional education (Teacher-centered)
Basis of instruction	Student outcomes (competencies)	Specific information to be covered
Pace of instruction	Learner sets own pace in meeting objectives	All proceed at pace determined by instructor
How to proceed from task to task	Master one task before moving to another	Fixed amount of time on each unit/module
Focus of instruction	Specific tasks included in role	Information that may or may not be part of role
Method of evaluation	Criterion referenced	Normative referenced

Source: Barbara Brunt, 2004.

Benefits of a competency-based approach include

- encouraging teamwork
- enhancing skills and knowledge
- increasing staff retention
- reducing staff anxiety
- increasing productivity
- improving nursing performance
- ensuring compliance with The Joint Commission (formerly known as the Joint Commission on Accreditation of Healthcare Organizations) standard that requires that all members of the staff are competent to fulfill their assigned responsibilities

The American Nurses Credentialing Center's (ANCC's) Magnet Recognition Program® objectives include promoting quality in a milieu that supports professional nursing practice and promoting positive patient outcomes. Designated hospitals' focus on outcomes and involvement of nurses in the decision-making process is consistent with the tenets of the CBE approach for individuals.

Evidence-based practice

Just as nurses are encouraged to use evidence-based data in their clinical practice, educators need to base their practice on current evidence. One way of determining if educators are fulfilling their responsibilities is to identify if competencies expected in their role are based on research or evidence of best practice.

According to Melnyk, evidence-based practice (EBP) is a problem-solving approach to clinical practice that incorporates the best evidence from well-designed studies, patient values, and patient preferences (Melnyk 2004). This definition not only incorporates research data, but also acknowledges patient values. The current focus on EBP has caused increased scrutiny of clinicians and their preparation.

Why is there such an emphasis on EBP? First and foremost, it can lead to better patient outcomes, but it also is a response to pressures for cost containment from payers and healthcare facilities. If better and more efficient treatments are incorporated into practice, then the length of stay should decrease, as well as overall costs.

Another reason for the focus on EBP is that consumers today are much more knowledgeable about treatment options. For example, it is not uncommon for patients to go to the Internet to find out more information about a specific disease, test, or treatment.

Ultimately, EBP provides opportunities for nurses to be more effective, and it acknowledges the value of nursing clinical judgment. Advantages of EBP are outlined in Figure 1.2.

FIGURE **1.2**   **Advantages of evidence-based practice**

Produces better patient outcomes and/or educational outcomes
Responds to pressure for cost containment from payers, healthcare facilities, and educational administrators
Acknowledges increased consumer awareness of treatment and care options and learners' savviness regarding educational strategies
Provides opportunities for nursing care and nursing education to be individualized, streamlined, more effective, and dynamic
Acknowledges the value of clinical judgment and critical thinking

Cileska et al. described a research study relating to the frequency with which staff nurses used various sources of knowledge (Cileska et al.2001). The top six sources were

1. experience
2. information learned in nursing school (although the average time since completion of a basic program was 18 years)
3. workplace sources
4. physician sources
5. intuition
6. past usual practice

Information from textbooks and journals ranked in the bottom six sources. The staff nurses were also asked to identify the one most common source from which they learned about research findings. Although 39% identified nursing journals, additional analyses showed that the primary journals the nurses read were not research journals but practice-focused journals published by professional nursing organizations.

Nursing is a complex profession, requiring a good knowledge base and critical-thinking skills. The function of nursing education is to produce a competent practitioner, adept in basic knowledge and with the ability to apply critical thinking. Nurse educators must address a wide range of skills and assist nurses in their integration of theory and practice. New approaches to education and practice should be based on research and evidence of best practices. NPD educators need to conduct research and utilize research findings on the best approaches to education and documentation of competency.

Competencies for nursing professional development educators

We need to ensure we are using evidence of best practices in all aspects of nursing, including education. Historically there has been little documentation of whether educators are using research-based methods or are competent to do the tasks with which they are entrusted.

There has been little research undertaken or articles published detailing specific competencies for NPD educators. Gordon and Franklin described how they developed an orientation to help prepare staff nurses for a clinical educator role (Gordon and Franklin 1993). However, the only topics that were outlined were principles of adult education and teaching strategies, performance checklists, needs assessments, and self-learning modules. As all staff educators know, the NPD educator role is more comprehensive than that.

Similarly, Kotecki and Eddy outlined how an orientation program was developed for staff development (SD) educators (Kotecki and Eddy 1994). The program identified only six competencies for this orientation, focusing on communication, clinical practice, needs assessments, developing an educational program, teaching, and determining if staff educational needs were being met. Although these are important competencies, they do not reflect the full scope of the nursing professional development educational role, as defined by the ANA's *Scope and Standards of Practice for Nursing Professional Development.*

Johnson detailed the development of competencies based upon the 1994 edition of the ANA's *Standards of Practice for Continuing Education and Staff Development*, and Benner's work reflected levels of practice and challenged educators to attain levels of excellence in practice (Johnson 2002). Use of these competencies involved a professional review process, components of peer input, self-evaluation, and portfolio development, but did not include research-based performance criteria. Vezina et al. described a competency-based orientation for clinical staff development educators involving an orientation manual, a guidebook, tracking forms, a teaching assessment, and a preceptor report (Vezina et al. 1996). Although these tools may help with educational competencies, they do not provide specific performance expectations for particular competencies.

Difference between NPD competencies and academic educator competencies

Nursing professional development activities exist in the domains of continuing education, staff development, and academic education. Academic education refers to those courses taken in colleges or universities after the basic nursing education program. Academic courses may or may not lead to a degree or completion of a certificate program.

Continuing education, staff development, and academic education overlap as nurses select the most effective way to meet their professional development needs and as educators engage in their practice roles. Academic education may be accessed to pursue a specific course of study for a degree or certificate or as individual courses through which to update one's knowledge in a particular area. Continuing education can be part of staff development or part of a formal academic program. Staff development can include continuing education activities, academic education, or both, as preparation for a particular role. This relationship is demonstrated in Figure 1.3 on page 12.

Although some aspects of the educational role are similar across all settings, differences exist in competencies expected in the NPD role and competencies expected of an academic educator in a university setting. The educational process does not change with the setting, so the competencies specific to assessment, planning, implementing, and evaluating educational activities would be the same. Some of the differences are noted below.

Academic educators most frequently are working with a group of students enrolled in an educational program over a preestablished period of time, usually a semester or quarter. These educators interact with the same group of students throughout that period, and can build on previous sessions as students progress through the curriculum. NPD educators frequently deal with participants in a single session, or for very short periods of time. This makes it more difficult to build on information provided in previous sessions.

FIGURE 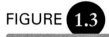 **1.3**   **Framework for Nursing Professional Development**

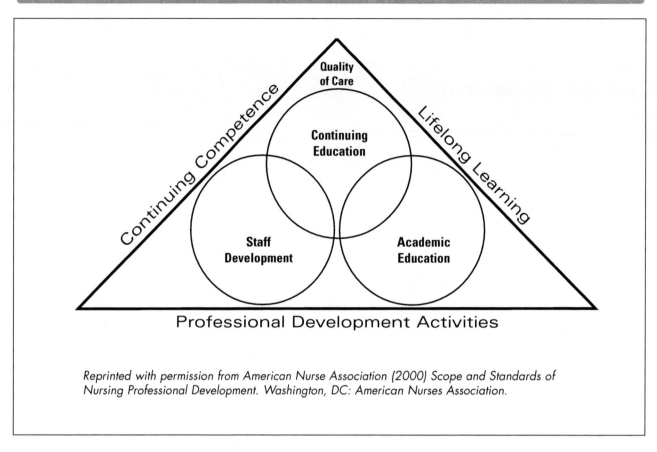

Reprinted with permission from American Nurse Association (2000) Scope and Standards of Nursing Professional Development. Washington, DC: American Nurses Association.

The National League for Nursing (NLN) identified core competencies of nurse educators. This effort arose from a Think Tank on Graduate Preparation for the Nurse Educator Role held in December 2001. Members of the Think Tank included faculty and administrators from associate degree, baccalaureate degree, and graduate nursing programs, as well as representatives from staff development and the higher education community. This group generated a list of eight competencies, with several ideas under each competency to further define its scope. Following the Think Tank, the Task Group on Nurse Educator Competencies began an extensive search of the literature to determine if the eight competencies were documented in evidence-based literature, or if there was a need to modify them. The final list had eight overall competencies, with 66 task statements identified to further describe the competencies. The overall competency statements are outlined in Figure 1.4 on page 13.

FIGURE **1.4** Core competencies of nurse educators

1. Facilitate learning
2. Facilitate learner development and socialization
3. Use assessment and evaluation strategies
4. Participate in curriculum design and evaluation of program outcomes
5. Function as change agents and leaders
6. Pursue continuous quality improvements in the nurse educator role
7. Engage in scholarship
8. Function within the educational environment

Source: Adapted from the National League for Nursing. (2005.) "Core competencies of nurse educators with task statements." New York: NLN. Retrieved on June 28, 2006, from www.nln.org/profdev/corecompetencies.pdf.

In many instances there are different expectations in the NPD role and academic role with respect to publishing. One of the task statements for the competency on facilitating learner development and socialization deals with dissemination of information through publications. The term "publish or perish" is frequently used with academic educators, who must publish to gain tenure. It is an expectation in many universities that faculty publish in peer-reviewed journals in their field. In most NPD educator roles, this is not a required competency.

One of the task statements under the competency of engaging in scholarship relates to demonstrating skills in proposal writing for initiatives that include, but are not limited to, research, resource acquisition, program development, and policy development. Grant writing is a task that is more commonly seen in academic education. Many NPD educators do not have any experience with grant writing and may not have the resources to develop expertise in that area. In many settings, academic educators are expected to write grants and receive funding for their research projects.

References

Alspach, J. G. 1995. *The Educational Process in Nursing Staff Development*. St. Louis: Mosby Year Book.

American Nurses Association. 2000. *Scope and Standards of Practice for Nursing Professional Development*. Washington, DC: American Nurses Association.

American Nurses Credentialing Center. 2006. "ANCC Magnet Recognition Program®." Silver Spring, MD: ANCC. Retrieved on June 29, 2006, from *www.nursingworld.org/ancc/magnet.html*.

Cileska, D. K., Pinelli, J., DiCenso, A., and Cullum, N. 2001. "Resources to enhance evidence-based nursing practice." *AACN Clinical Issues* 12 (4): 520–528.

Dickenson-Hazard, N. 2004. "Global health issues and challenges." *Journal of Nursing Scholarship* 36 (1): 6–10.

Gordon, B. N., and Franklin, E. M. 1993. "An orientation for inexperienced educators." *Journal of Nursing Staff Development* 9 (2): 75–77.

Johnson, S. 2002. "Development of educator competencies and the professional review process." *Journal for Nurses in Staff Development* 18 (2): 92–102.

Kelly-Thomas, K. J. 1998. *Clinical and Nursing Staff Development: Current Competence, Future Focus*. 2nd ed. Philadelphia: Lippincott, Williams & Wilkins.

Kotecki, C. N., and Eddy, J. R. 1994. "Developing an orientation program for a nurse educator." *Journal of Nursing Staff Development* 10 (6): 301–305.

Melnyk, B. M. 2004. "Integrating levels of evidence into clinical decision making." *Pediatric Nursing* 30 (4): 323–325.

National League for Nursing. 2005. "Core competencies of nurse educators with task statements." New York: NLN. Retrieved on June 28, 2006, from *www.nln.org/profdev/corecompetencies.pdf*.

National Nursing Staff Development Organization. 1999. "*Strategic Plan 2000*." Pensacola, FL: National Nursing Staff Development Organization.

Vezina, M., Chiang, J. J., Laufer, K., Garabedian, C., Padre, H., and Sanders, N. 1996. "Competency-based orientation for clinical nurse educators." *Journal of Nursing Staff Development* 12 (6): 311–313.

Developing educator competencies

Learning objective

After reading this chapter, the participant should be able to

- describe the research process used to develop the competencies and performance criteria

Performing a nursing professional development research study

Performance criteria for the comprehensive list of nursing professional development competencies, included in Appendix A, came from an extensive research study completed in three stages over a four-year period. Figure 2.1 on page 16 provides an overview of the entire study.

Origins of the competencies

The first stage built upon a Delphi research study on advanced practice competencies completed by the ANA Council on Continuing Education and Staff Development (CE/SD) and NNSDO in 1995. The goal of the Delphi technique is to reach consensus on a particular topic. A panel of experts gives individual feedback on a subject, which is then judged by the entire panel. The process is repeated, building on information obtained in each round, until some agreement is obtained. The study identified 63 advanced practice competencies in continuing education and staff development.

FIGURE **2.1** **Overview of the research study**

Starting point: *Advanced Practice Report* (NNSDO 1997), outlining 63 advanced practice competencies in continuing education and staff development
Development of a self-assessment tool with 116 basic and advanced competencies
Completion of a pilot study to validate a method to identify performance criteria for 10 competency statements
Nine additional studies completed to identify performance criteria for a total of 109 competency statements
Validation of survey results for 25 competencies by a group of academic educators
Consolidation and grouping of competencies and performance criteria using ANA standards, Harden's model, and Benner's framework
Testing of researcher's "novice" to "expert" categorization with a group of local and national staff development educators
Development of final Nursing Professional Development Educator Competency Tool

The author of this book added basic competencies derived from a review of the literature and 20 years of experience in staff development to create a self-assessment tool with 116 competency statements.

When individuals completing the self-assessment tool had questions about how they would know whether they had achieved a particular competency, the primary investigator (PI) identified the need for specific performance criteria.

Ongoing research

In the second stage of the study, the researcher eliminated some redundant competencies from the self-assessment tool and started with 109 competency statements, which were all classified as either objective or subjective. Quantitative research methods were used for the objective statements and qualitative methods were used for the subjective statements.

A pilot study was completed to validate the method used to identify performance criteria, and nine additional phases of stage 2 were completed to identify performance criteria for all 109 competencies. For each phase of this study, feedback was obtained from a random, stratified sample of nurses certified in Nursing Professional Development, as well as regional groups. A description of the method used for the pilot study and subsequent studies is outlined in the 2002 article in the *Journal for Nurses in Staff Development*.

These studies provided a comprehensive description of NPD competencies with specific performance criteria to determine whether an educator met those competencies. These studies established the validity and reliability of an extensive range of competency statements and accompanying performance criteria that could be used by NPD educators with a range of expertise, from novice to expert.

Validating the results

Stage 3 involved validating the results of the national and regional samples with a group of academic educators for 25 selected competencies and performance criteria. Nurse faculty members from a list of educators in NLN-accredited baccalaureate and masters nursing programs throughout the United States were invited to participate in an online survey.

This survey used the same Likert scale as the other phases. A Likert scale is a form of response scale commonly used with questionnaires. When responding to a Likert questionnaire item, respondents specify their level of agreement to a given statement. Results from this group were compared with the national sample of certified nurses and regional sample of NNSDO affiliates, to determine whether there were similarities in the competencies and performance criteria across different settings.

Refining the results

The final stage of this study refined the competency statements and performance criteria based on the feedback received in stages 2 and 3. The PI analyzed feedback from respondents to reduce duplication in the competency statements and further clarify performance criteria for the competencies.

The statements were consolidated into 72 competencies and were placed into a framework, which is described in Chapter 3. For any competency where there was a significant difference between the national and regional results, a small group of expert SD educators (the Executive Board of NNSDO) was asked to provide additional feedback. The result was a comprehensive, research-based tool to measure the competence of NPD educators.

The information obtained from this study may be applicable to educators in other disciplines and in other settings throughout the United States and the world. Others could replicate the method used in the research to identify performance criteria for other specialties.

References

Benner, P. 1984. *From Novice to Expert: Excellence and Power in Clinical Nursing Practice.* Menlo Park, CA: Addison-Wesley.

Brunt, B. A. 1999. *Competencies of Staff Development Educators: Personal Assessment of Competency.* Akron, OH: Summa Health System.

Brunt, B. A. 2002. "Identifying performance criteria for staff development competencies." *Journal for Nurses in Staff Development* 18(4): 213–217.

Brunt, B. A. 2005. "Identifying performance criteria for staff development competencies." Unpublished master's dissertation. University of Dundee, Scotland.

National Nursing Staff Development Organization. 1997. *Report of the Task Force on Advanced Practice in Nursing Continuing Education and Staff Development.* Pensacola, FL: NNSDO.

Creating a framework for educator competencies

Learning objective

After reading this chapter, the participant should be able to
- identify how the educational competencies fit with the ANA standards, Harden's outcome model, and Benner's novice-to-expert continuum

Key concepts

The following definitions of key concepts from the ANA's *Scope and Standards of Practice for Nursing Professional Development* are presented to guide the discussion in this chapter.

Continuing competence: Ongoing professional nursing competence according to level of expertise, responsibility, and domains of practice. The competence is evidenced by behavior based on beliefs, attitudes, and knowledge matched to and in the context of a set of expected outcomes, and it is defined by nursing scope of practice, policy, code of ethics, standards, guidelines, and benchmarks that ensure safe performance of professional activities.

Nursing professional development educator: A registered nurse whose practice is in nursing education and who facilitates lifelong learning in a variety of healthcare, educational, and academic settings.

Standards of nursing practice: Authoritative statements that describe a level of care or performance common to the profession of nursing and by which the quality of nursing practice can be judged and reassured.

Standards of professional performance: Authoritative statements that describe a competent level of behavior in the professional role, including activities related to quality of care, performance appraisal, education, collegiality, ethics, collaboration, research, and resource utilization.

Using ANA standards to build a framework

The ANA standards for nursing professional development that were published in 2000 can be used to provide a framework for the NPD competencies and performance criteria that were identified in the research studies. These standards are divided into six standards of practice and eight standards of professional performance.

Standards of practice
 1. Assessment
 2. Diagnosis
 3. Analysis to determine target audience and learner needs
 4. Identification of educational outcomes
 5. Planning
 6. Implementation and evaluation

Standards of professional performance

1. Quality of NPD practice

2. Performance appraisal

3. Education

4. Collegiality

5. Ethics

6. Collaboration and research

7. Management and resource utilization

8. Leadership

The standards and corresponding outcome criteria focus on competencies appropriate for NPD educators practicing in all settings.

The ANA standards are built on a framework of continuing competence. In the philosophy of NPD outlined in the standards, there were 13 belief statements that guided the development of the standards. Eight of the 13 belief statements had the word "competence" included in the statement. There is a great need for competent, committed, and creative educators prepared to facilitate diverse learners' educational achievements. The roles of NPD educators identified in the standards were educator, facilitator, change agent, consultant, researcher, and leader. Figure 3.1 outlines key components of each of these roles.

To evaluate whether NPD educators are meeting the standards, outcome assessments can be used to identify, define, and communicate the skills and qualities that NPD educators should possess.

FIGURE **3.1** **Roles of nursing professional development educators**

Educator role:
- Provide appropriate climate for learning
- Facilitate adult learning process
- Involve learners
- Ensure qualified faculty
- Evaluate activities and outcomes
- Use portfolio to document continuing competence
- Develop, plan, and present educational activities
- Encourage critical thinking and problem solving
- Maintain strong theory base

Facilitator role:
- Assist learners in identifying both their learning needs and the effective learning activities required to meet those needs
- Provide time for individuals to meet their educational needs or guide them to the appropriate resources
- Work with intra- or interdisciplinary teams to brainstorm and problem-solve
- Participate in strategic planning
- Serve as a role model for education
- Facilitate team building
- Foster a positive attitude about the benefits and opportunities of lifelong learning

Change agent role:
- Serve as a change agent at the organizational, community, state, national, or international level
- Facilitate the initiation of, adoption of, and adaptation to change
- Identify what changes should be made through leadership and participation in various activities such as committees, task forces, projects, and organizational strategic-planning meetings
- Influence the necessary policy, procedures, or legislation to create change

Consultant role:
- Assist with integration of new learning into the practice or educational environment
- Serve as a resource in assisting nurses to design needed educational experiences
- Provide access to experiences for groups, departments, organizations, and other social entities
- Assist individuals and groups with defining problems, identifying available internal and external educational resources, and selecting educational options
- Provide feedback to the learners and the organization related to the effectiveness of the learning and the learning activity

FIGURE 3.1   Roles of nursing professional development educators (cont.)

Researcher role:
- Design, create, and apply research
- Integrate relevant research outcomes into NPD activities
- Support integration of research into practice
- Help develop staff members' knowledge and skills in the research process
- Foster use of systematic evaluative research
- Evaluate outcomes of educational endeavors
- Track learner outcomes as profession moves to evidence-based practice
- Be active in research process as principal investigator, collaborator, or evaluator

Leader role:
- Provide and support organizational structures
- Manage overall program activities, including human and financial resources
- Use negotiation skills
- Communicate
- Demonstrate problem-solving skills
- Participate in activities external to organization
- Maintain appropriate competencies for role
- Maintain ethical principles

Outcomes should be expressed in such a way that they

- reflect the vision or mission of the institution
- are clear and unambiguous
- are specific and address defined areas of competence
- are manageable in terms of the number of outcomes
- are defined at an appropriate level of generality, assisting with the development of "enabling" outcomes
- indicate the relationship between different outcomes

Measuring outcomes

Harden and others proposed a three-circle model for assessing outcomes by classifying learner outcomes to evaluate performance (Harden et al. 1999). This model is based on the three dimensions of the work of a doctor, which also can be applied to the work of an NPD educator.

The inner circle represents what the educator is able to do, or "doing the right thing." It can be equated with technical intelligence, in line with Gardner's multiple intelligences model. The middle circle represents the way the educator approaches tasks, or "doing the thing right." This includes scientific understanding, ethics, decision-making, and analytical strategies, which comprise the academic, emotional, and analytical intelligences. The outer circle represents the development of the personal attributes of the educator, or "the right person doing it." This equates with the personal intelligences.

Harden's model acknowledges the need for a variety of teaching and assessment strategies to achieve the outcomes. For instance, approaches to learning that encourage reflective thinking can contribute to achievement of the learning outcomes in the middle circle. The focus on learning outcomes provides the framework that educators can use to determine whether they are meeting educational competencies.

Choosing a model

All the competencies and performance criteria developed from the research studies were put into Harden's outcome model and the educator roles identified in the *Scope and Standards of Practice for Nursing Professional Development* (ANA 2000). The roles identified by ANA in the standards of practice fit in well with Harden's inner circle ("doing the right thing"). The standards of professional performance fit into Harden's middle and outer circles. To further define the continuum of educational practice, the competencies within each category were ranked to differentiate levels of competence, using Benner's novice-to-expert theory.

Benner's novice-to-expert theory

Benner and others have done a significant amount of work on differentiating levels of competence (Benner et al. 1996). Benner's five-stage model of skill acquisition indicated that nurses progress through various stages of qualitatively different perceptions of their task as skills improve from a novice to expert level (see Figure 3.2.) A novice has no experience or background with the skills, and needs structure and specific guidelines for performance. Advanced beginners have some experience with the application of knowledge and skills, but still need considerable guidance. They have difficulty setting priorities and generally lack the flexibility of the more experienced nurse. Competent practitioners have a basic comfort level with the application of

FIGURE **3.2** **Skill expectations in Benner's novice-to-expert continuum**

Novice	No experience or background with the skill; needs structure and specific guidelines for performance
Advanced beginner	Some experience with application of knowledge and skill, but still needs considerable guidance; has difficulty setting priorities; lacks flexibility
Competent	Basic comfort level with application of knowledge and skill; conscious, deliberate problem solving; sets priorities; sees actions in terms of long-range goals/performance
Proficient	Comfortable enough with application of knowledge and skills to adjust priorities based on anticipated response; perceives situation as a whole; performance is guided by subtle nuances
Expert	Extensive background and mastery of application of knowledge and skill; intuitive grasp of the situation; able to adjust spontaneously as needed

knowledge and skills, and follow a conscious and deliberate problem-solving approach to their practice. They set priorities and see their actions in terms of long-range goals/performance. Proficient nurses are comfortable enough with the application of knowledge and skills to adjust priorities based on anticipated response. They perceive the situation as a whole, and their performance is guided by subtle nuances. Expert practitioners have an extensive background and mastery of the application of knowledge and skill, demonstrating an intuitive grasp of the situation, with the ability to adjust spontaneously as needed.

Ordering the competencies to reflect the novice-to-expert continuum

According to many authors, competency checklists can detect differences in novice, competent, and expert practitioners. To reflect this, the competencies were ordered in each section on a continuum from novice to expert expectations.

To determine how the competencies fit within Benner's framework, feedback was obtained from two pilot groups. One group was a local group of 19 educators with a range of experience from less than one month to 30 years. The other group was a national group of 25 educators with a range of experience from one year to 25 years. Participants in the pilot groups were asked to check the competencies they felt they had met and identify how many years they had been functioning as an NPD educator. Data did not yield consistency in the number of years to achieve the competency. However, responses of all members of the pilot group were ordered based on the number of individuals who had met that competency. The highest number would indicate basic competencies, since more individuals had met that competency, whereas the lower numbers would indicate more advanced competencies. Feedback from those groups was used to refine the placements of the competency statements within each of the role categories from the scope and standards of practice.

Data was sorted by years, patterns were analyzed, and the criteria under each of the roles in Harden's "doing the right thing" category were reordered based on participant feedback. There was much less variability in the categories of "doing the right thing" and the "right person doing it." This may be explained by the fact that the criteria in these categories are more general and personal attributes, rather than role-related.

The final list of competencies by category is listed on the next page. For specific performance criteria for each of the statements, refer to the Nursing Professional Development Educator Competency Assessment Tool, included in the Appendix.

Final list of competencies by category

What educators are able to do: "Doing the right thing"
Educator role

1. Designs and revises educational activities
2. Uses a variety of teaching strategies and audiovisuals
3. Uses and evaluates material resources and facilities
4. Conducts needs assessment using a variety of strategies
5. Involves learners in assessment of needs and identification of outcomes
6. Determines and revises priorities for scheduled and unscheduled educational activities
7. Evaluates effectiveness and outcomes of educational endeavors
8. Coordinates complex educational offerings
9. Selects appropriate teaching strategies to facilitate behavioral change
10. Develops curriculums (classes or courses around a common theme)
11. Adjusts content and teaching strategy during presentation based on learners' reactions
12. Creates and applies newer educational methodologies
13. Uses appropriate measurement methods to assess and document competence of personnel
14. Possesses expert knowledge of how to teach within organizational culture
15. Measures and communicates return on investment (ROI)

Researcher role

16. Supports integration of research into practice
17. Incorporates research findings from a variety of disciplines into programs
18. Accesses resources needed to facilitate research
19. Develops and conducts research

Facilitator role

20. Involves the client in defining problems and seeking solutions
21. Collaborates within and across organization
22. Facilitates the adult learning process, creating a climate conducive to learning and a good relationship with learners
23. Identifies internal and external resources available for staff

24. Develops sponsor relationships with business and industry

25. Develops links with academia and service

Consultant role

26. Participates in committees, task forces, projects, etc.

27. Networks within and outside nursing

28. Provides technical assistance to clients

29. Coaches and provides feedback to improve performance

30. Differentiates educational problems from system problems

31. Uses consultation skills internally and externally

32. Consults on performance problems

33. Conducts focus groups

Leader role

34. Maintains required documentation and recordkeeping system

35. Facilitates team-building

36. Evaluates overall educational program effectiveness

37. Develops standards for educational practice in own setting

38. Develops or provides input into annual budget

39. Uses appropriate measurement tools and methods in quality-improvement activities

40. Applies skill in strategic planning

41. Markets the SD/CE program

42. Calculates risks and benefits of innovations

43. Writes grant proposals or participates in grant-writing process

Change agent role

44. Facilitates change

45. Serves as a change agent

How educators approach practice: "Doing the thing right"

46. Maintains confidentiality

47. Promotes a safe and healthy work environment

48. Uses principles from theories of adult learning; organizational development; and system, change, and quality management

49. Integrates ethical principles in all aspects of practice

50. Demonstrates expertise in use of computers

51. Maintains educational standards

52. Communicates effectively with all levels of organization

53. Ensures educational programs are congruent with organizational mission and goals

54. Maintains flexibility when managing multiple roles and responsibilities

55. Interprets and communicates across boundaries

56. Accesses information external to organization

57. Communicates impact of new educational strategies to others

58. Demonstrates awareness of historical and emerging trends

59. Fosters use of systematic analysis of issues

60. Mentors other professionals

61. Critically processes information and problem-solves

62. Produces desired outcomes relevant to organization

63. Develops proactive educational policies and procedures for organization

64. Functions within the political climate of the organization

65. Publishes information that can be used by other educators

Development of individual attributes: "Right person doing it"

66. Maintains educational or clinical competencies appropriate for role

67. Promotes concept of lifelong learning

68. Establishes credibility with other professionals

69. Serves as role model for education

70. Seeks opportunities to develop the various SD roles as defined by the ANA

71. Participates in activities external to practice setting

72. Sees beyond role-established barriers

With the comprehensive list of competencies just listed, there are criteria for staff development educators at any point on the continuum from novice to expert practitioner. Implementation of the competencies and corresponding performance criteria can be tailored to the individual's staff development practice. This chapter describes the framework for the competencies and the rationale for the ordering of competencies in each section; practical application can be found in later chapters.

References

American Nurses Association. 2000. *Scope and Standards of Practice for Nursing Professional Development*. Washington, DC: ANA.

Benner, P. 1984. *From Novice to Expert: Excellence and Power in Clinical Nursing Practice*. Menlo Park, CA: Addison-Wesley.

Benner, P., Tanner, C. A., and Chesla, C. A. 1996. *Expertise in Nursing Practice: Caring, Clinical Judgment and Ethics*. New York: Springer Publishing.

Brunt, B. A. 2005. "Identifying performance criteria for staff development competencies." Unpublished master's dissertation. University of Dundee, Scotland.

Gardner, H. 1983. *Frames of Mind*. New York: Basic Books.

Harden, R. M., Crosby, J. R., Davis, M. H., and Friedman, M. 1999. "Part 5: From competency to meta-competency: A model for the specification of learning outcomes." In *AMEE Medical Education Guide No 14: Outcome based education*. Dundee, Scotland: Centre for Medical Education, 37–45.

Methods to validate competencies

Learning objective

After reading this chapter, the participant should be able to

- list at least four methods to validate competence

How do you measure competence?

There are numerous issues related to assessing and validating competence. Educators struggle with the following questions:

1. Who is responsible for assessing and documenting competence?
2. What tools can be used to validate competence?
3. How do you use competencies to evaluate performance?
4. How do you differentiate levels of competence?

Much of the discussion related to continued competence is focused on whose responsibility it is to assess and document competence. The ANA Code of Ethics discusses the individual nurse's personal responsibility to maintain competence in practice, and the ANA nursing scope and standards document reiterates the need for nurses to provide competent care and attain a level of knowledge and competency that reflects current nursing practice. The ANA scope and standards document for NPD is based on the concept of continuing competence.

Organizations must ensure that all staff members providing patient care are appropriately educated and competent to fulfill their job responsibilities. Hospitals have an ethical and legal responsibility to make certain that the healthcare provided by its personnel meets acceptable standards. To ensure the ongoing competence of employees, employers carry out the requirements of the Joint Commission on Accreditation of Healthcare Organizations (JCAHO) and other accrediting bodies. Educators assist with this responsibility by developing competency assessment and/or development programs. NPD educators often write competencies and validate both initial and continued competence.

Professional associations have a responsibility to set standards of performance and guidelines for safe practice. Competency validation is a partnership with the individual, agency, and professional association, as shown in Figure 4.1.

FIGURE **4.1** **Competency validation partnership**

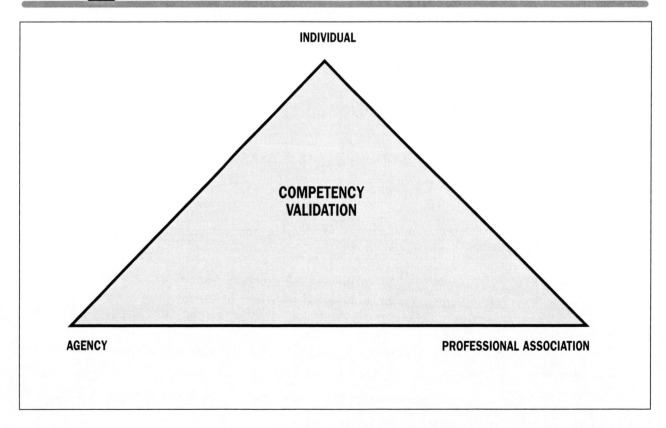

Competency checklists

Competency checklists are one way of validating competence. Checklists must clearly identify expectations and should be completed by staff members who know how to use them. Criteria for safe, effective performance must be clearly defined, and all parties involved in the evaluation process must have a common understanding of the criteria and the basis for assigning ratings. Research has shown that making direct observations using precise measurement criteria in checklists, with immediate feedback on performance, is more effective than the traditional evaluation of clinical skills using subjective rating forms. The format for skills checklists may vary, but most of them contain similar information. Characteristics of competency checklists are identified below.

Characteristics of competency checklists

- Learner oriented
- Focus on behaviors
- Measurable
- Criteria validated by experts
- Specific enough to avoid ambiguity

Most checklists use a "met" and "not met" format, include an area for comments, and evaluate a single occurrence. One drawback with checklists is that they do not identify whether the observed behavior is a persistent one that is representative of the situation being observed, or whether it is a snapshot of performance at a particular point in time. It is also important to assess clinical competence in the context of the "real" situation. Each institution determines how many and how often competency checklists should be used.

Some competency checklists have a self-assessment portion as part of the checklist. The self-assessment can give the evaluator an idea of the perceived skill level of the individual, although that can never take the place of validating the competency. Individuals may have different perceptions of their abilities, which may or may not be consistent with the evaluator's perceptions. For instance, some individuals might indicate they need practice because, even though they are very familiar and competent with that skill, they are not familiar with the institution's policy and procedure, while others might indicate they need practice because they have done it only once during their career. All required skills must be validated, regardless of the individual's assessment of his or her ability.

Other tools to validate competence

It is important to realize that there are numerous ways to validate competence. One of the most common is the competency checklist, but there are many other methods for validating competence.

Post-tests

Post-tests are one method to document cognitive knowledge and are sometimes used to document competence. Specifically, a post-test can be used to document basic knowledge so participants don't have to take a course or program when they can show they have the basic knowledge required in that course. For instance, some computer-based programs give participants the opportunity to complete the post-test first, and if they achieve a satisfactory score on the post-test, they don't have to complete the program.

Tests can include a videotape or audiotape scenario, a live simulation, or printed or projected still pictures requiring a response from the individual. A crossword puzzle or word game can also serve as a post-test.

Case studies

Case studies can also be used to validate competence. In this format, individuals describe how they would provide education for a specific student or how they would deal with a particular scenario presented to them. See the following for an example of an educational case study.

Sample educational case study

Situation: You are teaching a mandatory session on a new model of care delivery to a large group of students at your institution. You have incorporated a variety of teaching strategies and an opening exercise to get everyone engaged in the topic. There is one learner who is being vocal about not wanting to attend the session and is questioning your ability to teach the content. The learner will not participate in the exercise and, in front of the entire group, loudly questions why this session is mandatory, as well as your authority to teach this.

1. What strategies can you use to deal with this difficult student?
2. What adult learning strategies are appropriate for this situation?

Simulated events

Simulated events, such as mock codes, can be used to validate competency. Set up a room with a simulated patient who needs cardiopulmonary resuscitation, or a room that has numerous breaks in infection control techniques, and then have participants identify all the things that are not correct. Some schools use volunteers as simulated patients on which staff can perform assessments or demonstrate various noninvasive clinical skills. Several companies have mannequins available that can simulate a variety of situations requiring interventions.

Observations of daily work

An **observation of daily work** is another method of validating competence, often used in performance evaluations and with peer review or 360-degree evaluations. The 360-degree evaluation incorporates feedback from a variety of individuals who interact with an individual, including the manager, peers, and individuals reporting to them, and so on. The use of different sources of information and different measures to evaluate competence increases validity.

Differentiating competencies and performance

Is there a difference between competence and performance? These terms are often used interchangeably in the literature. One way of differentiating these two concepts is to define competence as what a person knows and can do under ideal circumstances, while performance focuses on actual situated behavior, i.e., what is actually done in the real-life context. If competence is causally related to performance, then the development of a competency should lead to increased effectiveness. However, one often observes a skill that is correlated with effective performance but that does not cause that performance.

For example, participants who are good at memorizing and writing may do well on tests, but that does not necessarily mean they will function more effectively in the clinical area. In developing training programs, the educator should remember that the employer judges competence of participants based on their ability to perform.

The goal of nursing education is to facilitate the transition of knowledge from the classroom to a variety of clinical experiences in a complex society with continually changing demographics, increased technology, and diminished resources. NPD educators are challenged to use educational strategies to enhance student learning while also promoting clinical competency.

Differentiating levels of competence

Benner's work on differentiating levels of competence was described in Chapter 3. Although many authors have attempted to reflect differences in the level of practice, few have developed tools with specific criteria for each level. Levels of performance are often differentiated by the ability to analyze and synthesize information.

Strategies that can be used to evaluate the level of competence include the following:

- Case studies can be used to evaluate critical thinking skills, as can open-ended questions to elicit feedback on thought processes.

- Mind mapping and concept mapping are other strategies that can be used to identify and correlate multiple aspects of a concept or problem. Both of these formats are nonlinear outlines or graphic representations of concepts or problems.

Learners begin by creating a colored image that represents the topic in the center of the paper. The next step is a "mind dump," in which participants write down all ideas related to the topic on a large piece of paper. Self-sticking notes may be used to jot down ideas and affix them to the paper. Participants can rearrange and cluster ideas in various configurations before settling on the most useful arrangement.

This chapter outlined various methods of validating competence, and included information on whose responsibility it is to develop competence. Descriptions of various tools to document competence and a discussion of the difference between competence and performance were provided, as well as suggestions for ways to differentiate levels of competence.

References

American Nurses Association. 2000. *Scope and Standards of Practice for Nursing Professional Development.* Washington, DC: ANA.

American Nurses Association. 2001. *Code of Ethics for Nurses with Interpretive Statements.* Washington, DC: ANA.

American Nurses Association. 2004. *Nursing: Scope and Standards of Practice.* 3rd ed. Washington, DC: ANA.

Brunt, B. A. 2004. "What is competency validation?" In *Competency Management System: A Toolkit for Validation and Assessment.* Marblehead, MA: HCPro.

SECTION II

Applications of the competencies to practice

This section provides examples of how the competencies can be used and applied in the practice setting in a variety of roles. Chapters in this section cover using the checklist as a self-assessment tool, to develop criterion-based position descriptions, to create an orientation for a new educator, for performance appraisals or professional development plans, and for a professional portfolio, as well as suggestions for documenting cultural competence.

Self-assessment

Learning objective

After reading this chapter, the participant should be able to

- complete a self-assessment using the checklist

Since the roles of NPD educators vary based on the size and type of organization, competencies can be selected to accurately reflect the NPD role in various settings. Not all of the competencies and performance criteria included in this book will be applicable to all NPD educators. Individuals can select the competencies that are appropriate for their current roles and responsibilities. With today's emphasis on professional accountability, it is critical that NPD educators, regardless of their role, demonstrate their competence and have a method to do so.

Using the checklist as a self-assessment tool

Practicing educators or individuals new to an educational role can use the tool in the Appendix as a self-assessment. This tool provides an overview of all aspects of the educational role, and can be tailored to the individual. For example, if an educator is in a setting that does not require research as part of the educational role, that competency can be ignored. Having specific performance criteria identified for each competency can assist educators to determine whether they have achieved that competency.

What should be assessed?

Educators' self-assessments should be tied to their setting's organizational goals. What do the educators need to learn or do that is not already part of their practice to more efficiently and effectively meet the goals of the organization? Relating aspects of NPD practice to organizational goals can help identify the value of education.

The tool may also assist educators in identifying where they are on the novice-to-expert continuum. Since the competencies in each subcategory are ranked in order from novice to expert, educators who meet the competencies at the end of each role or category may be practicing at a more advanced level.

Suggestions for using the self-assessment tool

Questions to ask when completing a self-assessment:

- Which of the skills are required in my current role or will be required in my new role?

- For each of those skills, can I provide examples of how I met the individual performance criteria?

- Are there some competencies where I met some but not all of the performance criteria listed?

- What experiences do I need to seek out to develop additional skills for a particular competency?

Be honest with yourself

Information derived from the self-assessment can be private and does not need to be shared with others. The educator completing the self-assessment should answer the questions honestly and use the information obtained as a guide in seeking additional experiences to meet identified needs.

Please note that even the most experienced educators will not be proficient in all the competencies listed. The number of competencies listed on the tool should not overwhelm new educators. This is designed as a tool to provide information for future learning opportunities.

■

Criterion-based position descriptions

Learning objective

After reading this chapter, the participant should be able to
- develop an educator position description specific to the setting

Developing position descriptions

Many regulatory agencies require organizations to have criterion-based position descriptions for staff, and the NPD competencies tool can be used to outline basic competencies and criteria that need to be included in a particular role.

Facilities can use the evidence-based data in the tool to write position descriptions. Since it provides a comprehensive classification of NPD competencies, it can be used for a variety of positions and in various settings. For example, the roles and responsibilities of a one-person staff development department in a small hospital would be different than those of a 10-person staff development department in a large teaching hospital in a healthcare system. The competencies and criteria can be selected to fit multiples roles.

Before writing a position description

The qualifications for being an NPD educator vary from setting to setting and are contingent on the roles and responsibilities of the department. There are various questions to consider before writing a position description, such as the following:

- What is the organization's philosophy, mission, vision, and values?
- Where does education fit within the organization?
- What are the goals and objectives of the education department?
- Is the organization a single entity or part of a larger healthcare system?
- What services does the education department provide (e.g., orientation, inservices, continuing education)?
- What are the reporting relationships?
- What educational qualifications are required for the position?
- What skills are required for the position?
- What is the organizational structure (e.g., centralized, decentralized, or a combination)?

The structure of an education department will guide the development of position descriptions, since educators may function differently in centralized versus decentralized or combination structures. In centralized models, staff development activities are performed by a core team of educators reporting to a single director. Decentralized models locate the responsibility for staff development at the level of the nursing department, a subdivision of that department, or at the unit level.

One form of a decentralized structure involves placing the responsibility for nursing staff development within a central nursing administration, with educators assigned to specific units. A second form may have some nurse educators assigned to a centralized nursing staff development program and others attached to various clinical divisions within the nursing services department. The most extreme form of decentralization places all responsibilities for staff development on individual nursing units.

The combination approach uses portions of both the centralized and decentralized structures to maximize their advantages and minimize their disadvantages.

Advantages and disadvantages of staff development structures are listed in Figure 6.1.

FIGURE **6.1** **Advantages and disadvantages of staff development structures**

	Advantages	**Disadvantages**
Centralized	Coordination of resources	Centralized decision-making
	Uniformity in implementing standards	Unresponsive to unit needs
	Coordination of regulatory and agency-required programming	Lack of coordination between general and unit programs
	Comprehensive and collaborative orientation activities	Lack of identity with specific areas
	Consistent education content and teaching methods	Dissatisfaction of educators with role
	More efficient use of educators	Possible reduced autonomy
	Support services readily available	Potential loss of clinical skills of educators
Decentralized	Educational needs more easily identified	Coordination may be ineffective or inefficient
	Increased opportunity for feedback and application	Duplication of education and efforts of personnel
	Increased educational leadership and involvement in departments	Inconsistent education and teaching methods
	Programming implemented in a timely manner	Lack of support services
	More flexibility in educational programming	Inadequate or inconsistent recordkeeping
	Educators seen as clinical experts	Educators may be used for service
Combination	Identification of individual unit needs	Cost of managing both designs may increase staffing
	Timely response to both centralized and decentralized education	Educators may lose sight of overall staff development goals
	Use of clinical experts for unit-based programming	
	Increased flexibility	
	Availability of support services	
	Coordination to reduce duplication and inappropriate use of resources	
	Collegial support for all educators	

Source: Brunt, B.A. (1998) "Structure and process: New models of nursing and clinical staff development." In K. J. Kelly-Thomas. *Clinical and Nursing Staff Development: Current Competence, Future Focus.* 2nd ed. Philadelphia: Lippincott, Williams & Wilkins. Reproduced with permission.

Once the questions are answered, then the competencies can be used as a framework to either develop the position descriptions or ensure that the essential competencies are identified in the position descriptions. Sample position descriptions for a staff development instructor and a director of nursing education and staff development are included as Exhibits 6.1 and 6.2.

> **TIP** | Develop position descriptions to include specific competencies/expectations in the educator/administrator role in your setting.

EXHIBIT **6.1** **Sample position description for staff development instructor**

Summa Health System Hospitals
Position Description

Title:	Staff Development Instructor (535)	Approvals	
Incumbent:		Incumbent _____ Date _____	
Reports to:	Director of Nursing Education and Staff Development	Supervisor _____ Date _____	
Department:	Staff Development (79151)	Administration _____ Date _____	
Function:	Staff Development Instructor	Human Resources _____ Date _____	
Date:	June, 2000	Position Code _____535_____	

Summary of Position

BASIC FUNCTION: Designs, organizes, implements, and evaluates educational programs (orientations, continuing education, and inservices) that facilitate the professional growth, skill development, competency, and attainment of standards of care for direct care providers within the following departments: Department of Patient Care Services and Ambulatory Care Services.

These programs will be developed, implemented, and evaluated using nursing theory, nursing clinical expertise, standards of practice, and adult education principles.

Dimensions of Position

Staff Development Instructors (5.5 FTE) are accountable for and impact the following:

Summa Health System Hospitals

Provision of educational support for:

FTE = 1,794 (1,279 RNs, 234 LPNs, 126 administrative associates [AA], 105 nursing assistants, and 50 environmental support associates)

Number of education activities processed:
- 12–14 RN/LPN orientations per year
- 12–14 Nursing Assistant (NA) orientations per year
- 12–14 Administrative Associate (AA) orientations per year
- 24–48 BLS/ACLS classes per year
- 631.8 (+) nursing contact hours per year
- 100–264 write and revise the Department of Patient Care Services policies and procedures
- 3–12 IV courses per year
- 6–10 Preceptor courses per year
- 12–14 Delegation classes per year
- 12 EKG classes per year (as needed)

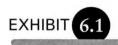

EXHIBIT 6.1

Sample position descriptions for staff development instructor (cont.)

- 12 Blood Glucose testing (BGT) classes per year (and individual competency as needed)
- 10+ Non Violent Crises Intervention (NVCI) Certification/Recertification classes per year
- 6 Neonatal Resuscitation (NRP) classes per year
- 4 Med/Surg curriculums per year
- 3–4 Critical Care curriculums per year
- 6 (+) OB EKG Classes/year
- 4 Behavioral Health curriculums per year
- 4 Women's Health updates per year
- Community professional workshops
    a) Addiction Conference
    b) Ambulatory Conference
    c) Joe Harp Critical Care Conference
    d) Oncology Symposium
    e) Stroke Workshop
    f) Women's Health Workshop
    g) Advanced Medical/Surgical Workshop
- 2 + Basic Fetal Monitoring courses per year
- Inservices: topics vary depending on Quality Improvement issues, new equipment, and new policies and procedures
    - Inservices are mainly done on the unit 1:1 for 38 clinical areas and other areas as deemed appropriate.
- 2 + Advanced Fetal Monitoring Principles + Practice Workshops/ per year
- PRN Fetal Monitoring updates as needed
- 3–12 Transfer and Transport classes for environmental support associates

Direct Management Reporting Leaderships

Staff Development Instructors report directly to the Director of Nursing Education and Staff Development.

Indirect/Functional Management Reporting Relationships

Staff Development instructors also collaborate with Unit Manager, other Directors of Patient Care, and Clinical Services.

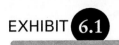

EXHIBIT **6.1** **Sample position descriptions for staff development instructor (cont.)**

KEY RESULT AND ACCOUNTABILITY AREAS

Note: The following key result and accountability areas will be carried out in a manner fully consistent with the Summa mission, values, and philosophies.

Common/Generic key results and accountability areas essential for position

1. **Planning and organizing**
   The incumbent must facilitate learning/educational programs/activities for the Department of Patient Care Services and Ambulatory Care Services. This position collaborates and coordinates orientations, inservices and continuing education/staff development programs with nursing directors, nursing managers, nursing staff, hospital departments, and community representatives.

2. **Managing and leading people**
   The incumbent designs, implements and evaluates education programs that assist nursing personnel to achieve competency and deliver safe care based on standards of practice.
   This position models professional roles and behaviors that assist nursing personnel to acquire competency, knowledge, and clinical skills.

3. **Managing and controlling financial resources**
   The incumbent prepares budgets and workshop cost analysis forms related to specific educational activities/programs for incorporation in the department's budget.

4. **Performance improvement**
   The incumbent compiles statistics and written documentation on mandatory educational activities and correlates stats to strategic goals, department and agency guidelines, standards of practice, and Providership regulation. This position demonstrates a philosophy of continual improvement by consistently evaluating need for specific educational activities, analyzing the best method of delivering education to customers, and actively participates in quality improvement activities/teams.

5. **Service quality**
   The incumbent is also responsible for identifying the direct and indirect groups served by Department of Patient Services and Ambulatory Services and Nursing Education, determining appropriate products and services that are based upon groups served needs, measuring group's satisfaction, and developing actions that continually improve services. Groups served include employees, managers, executives, and physicians. Indirect groups served include patients, Board members, and professional community.

6. **Relationships with managers, peers, etc.**
   The incumbent is responsible for developing and maintaining open, honest, and mutually beneficial relationships with his or her manager, fellow managers, staff, and the departments to which he/she provides service. Relationships will be maintained in a manner consistent with Summa's mission, values, and philosophies.

EXHIBIT 6.1 **Sample position descriptions for staff development instructor (cont.)**

7. **Supporting diversity**
The incumbent is responsible for ensuring a work environment within his or her department that promotes and embraces diversity. The incumbent formulates educational programs and/or materials that assist personnel to care for patients across age-specific populations and across various cultural and religious groups.

8. **Development of self and others**
The incumbent is responsible for continued self-development through attendance at various Summa-sponsored management development programs, professional seminars, and conferences. Also, the incumbent is responsible for ensuring the continued development of staff.

9. **Communication**
The incumbent is responsible for ensuring excellent open communications within the department. This includes attendance at regular staff meetings, and preparation and distribution of minutes, reports, and other means to keep the department informed on a timely basis. The incumbent will communicate effectively with his or her manager, peers, other members of Summa Management Team, employees, and outside customers.

10. **Regulatory compliance**
The incumbent is responsible for complying with regulatory and accreditation requirements through completion of Summa's mandatory organizational education, JCAHO, Code of Conduct, and compliance training. Incumbent also responsible for adherence to Summa's mandatory organizational educational education requirements, JCAHO standards, Code of Conduct, and Compliance Plan in daily activities and work processes. Incumbent also responsible for complying with professional standards of practice and Ohio Nurses Association Continuing Education Providership.

Specific key results and accountability areas essential for position

Insert the 5 or 6 key result and accountability areas in this section. These should be the major categories of responsibility for this position. Under each heading, summarize in 3-4 sentences the accountability and expectation.

1. **Orientation**
The incumbent plans, organizes, implements, and evaluates clinical orientation for all levels of nursing personnel, both at the individual and departmental levels.

2. **Policy & Procedure Writing**
The incumbent writes and revises the Department of Patient Care Services policies and procedures. The incumbent assists nursing units to write and revise their department/unit policies and procedures.

3. **Continuing Education**
The incumbent writes continuing nursing education (CE) applications for selected educational programs following the Ohio Nurses Association CE Providership Guidelines.

     Competencies for Staff Educators: Tools to Evaluate and Enhance Nursing Professional Development

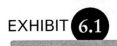

EXHIBIT 6.1 **Sample position descriptions for staff development instructor (cont.)**

4. <u>BLS / ACLS / Crisis Intervention, Neonatal Resuscitation and Fetal Monitoring</u>
The incumbent prepares and teaches in the mandatory BLS/ACLS/Crisis Intervention, Neonatal Resuscitation, and Fetal Monitoring courses.

5. <u>Patient Education</u>
The incumbent prepares and/or assists clinical nursing personnel to develop/purchase materials to teach patients/populations of patients.

6. <u>Curriculums/Inservices</u>
The incumbent, in collaboration with nursing managers, nursing staff peers, and other hospital departments, designs, organizes, implements, and evaluates curriculums and inservices that assist nursing personnel to care for various populations of patients.

Note: The above stated duties are intended to outline those functions typically performed by the incumbent in this position. This description of duties is not intended to be all-inclusive or to limit the discretionary authority of supervisors to assign additional tasks of a similar nature or level of responsibility.

BACKGROUND, EXPERIENCE, AND EDUCATION

1. **Experience:**
Three (3) years professional RN experience and
One (1) year formal teaching experience

2. **Education and training**
Current license to practice nursing.
Masters degree in Nursing or Education
OR
Baccalaureate degree in Nursing with definite plans to complete Master's Degree in Nursing or Education

3. **Skills/competencies**
Excellent verbal and written communication skills
Ability to work collaboratively with various levels of nursing personnel, Medical Staff, Community Representatives.

4. **Age-related competency**
The incumbent will have the ability to effectively interact with patients/customers (i.e., neonates/newborns, children, adolescents, young adults, middle-aged adults, and geriatric adults, as applicable) with the understanding of their needs for self-respect and dignity.

5. **Other qualifications**
Ability to use computer and audiovisual equipment.

EXHIBIT **6.1** **Sample position descriptions for staff development instructor (cont.)**

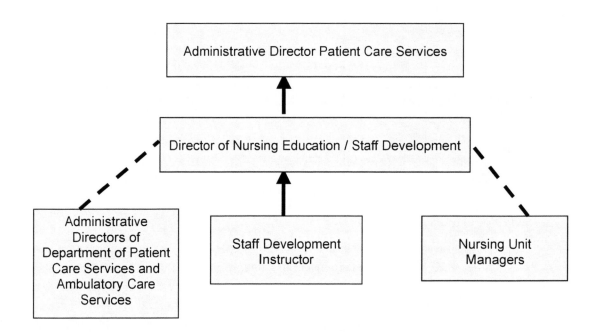

SUMMA HEALTH SYSTEM HOSPITALS ORGANIZATION CHART

The organizational chart should accurately reflect the reporting relationships within the department. It should include what position this position reports to and any direct or indirect reports to this position.

Administrative Director Patient Care Services

Director of Nursing Education / Staff Development

Administrative Directors of Department of Patient Care Services and Ambulatory Care Services

Staff Development Instructor

Nursing Unit Managers

© 2000. Summa Health System. Reproduced with permission

EXHIBIT 6.2 **Sample position description for director of nursing education and staff development**

SUMMA HEALTH SYSTEM
- POSITION DESCRIPTION -

Title: Director, Nursing Education & Staff Development   Approvals

Incumbent: Barbara Brunt   Incumbent: _____

Date: _____

Reports to: Administrative Director, Patient Care Services   Supervisor: _____

Date: _____

Department: Staff Development

Administration: _____ Date: _____

Function: Nursing Education / Staff Development   Human Resources:_____ Date: _____

Date Updated: 8/17/05   Position Code: _____

Updated By: Barbara Brunt, MA, MN, RN, BC

Summary of Position (Briefly explain the purpose of this position)

Facilitates, directs, and coordinates the designing, planning, implementing, and evaluating of educational programs, activities, and services for the Department of Patient Care Services and Ambulatory Care Services. Ensures that such programs/services promote professional growth of personnel, competency of personnel, learning needs of patients and families, and attainment of hospital's strategic goals. Ensures that educational programs/services are consistent with criteria and standards of care established by licensing and accrediting bodies and professional organizations. Coordinates orientations/clinical experiences for all nursing and medical assistant students coming to Summa Health System Hospitals. Coordinates tracking of hospital-wide educational/safety programs

Dimensions of Position (Summarize the key statistics for which this position is directly and indirectly responsible, e.g., FTEs, operating expenses, revenues, volume indicators)

Summa Health System Hospitals
-   FTEs: 13.5 (Total)
-   7.3 Staff Development Instructors
-   1 Coordinator, Educational Facilities.
-   4.2 Clerk Typists
-   1 Senior Administrative Secretary

Provides education for 1,808 (1,320 RNs, 205 LPNs, 147 Unit Secretaries, 136 Nursing Assistants/Support Associates)

Capital Budget: $51,193 for 2005   Operating Budgets: $641,342 (labor, materials & supplies)
      Revenue: varies $10,000-$20,000

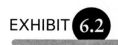

EXHIBIT 6.2 **Sample position description for director of nursing education and staff development (cont.)**

Direct Management Reporting Relationships (Indicate the title that this position reports to as well as the various titles reporting directly to this position)

Director of Nursing Education and Staff Development reports directly to the Administrative Director of Patient Care Services.
Reporting directly to the Manager of Nursing Education and Staff Development are:
1. 79151 Staff Development Instructors
2. 79181 Clerk typists and Senior Administrative Secretaries
3. 75611 Coordinator of Educational Facilities

Indirect/Functional Management Reporting Relationships (Indicate any position to which this position has an indirect reporting relationship as well as the position(s) over which this job has indirect management authority).

KEY RESULT AND
ACCOUNTABILITY AREAS

Note: The following key results and accountability areas will be carried out in a manner fully consistent with the Summa Mission, values, and philosophies.

Common/Generic key results and accountability areas essential for position

1. Planning and organizing
This position must plan and organize all activities under his/her control in an effective manner. This includes preparing departmental tactical and strategic plans as well as designing appropriate organizational structures for areas of responsibility. This responsibility also includes organizing and delegating work in an effective manner, for establishing appropriate time frames for completion of work, and for providing the necessary leadership to ensure effective work results.

2. Managing and leading people
This position selects, develops, and counsels the function's employee staff consistent with good human resources management practices and creates a work environment that encourages and allows participation in order to promote retention, productivity, employee safety, and a quality, customer-oriented employee staff. The incumbent plans and conducts staff meetings ensuring needs are anticipated and implementation of department tactics are discussed and implementation planned.

3. Managing and controlling financial resources
The incumbent plans, prepares, implements, monitors, and controls assigned areas' operational and capital budgets to ensure sound fiscal management consistent with the goals of Summa Health System.

EXHIBIT 6.2 **Sample position description for director of nursing education and staff development (cont.)**

4. Performance improvement

The incumbent is directly responsible for ensuring that his/her department adopts a Total Quality Improvement approach to its work that includes employee empowerment, managing with data, a philosophy of continual improvement, a customer-driven attitude, and a work methodology that maximizes error prevention. This responsibility includes developing and maintaining a complete quality monitoring system throughout his or her department.

5. Service quality

The incumbent is also responsible for identifying the direct and indirect groups served by the Department of Patient Care Services, Ambulatory Services, and Nursing Education, determining appropriate products and services that are based upon groups' served needs, measuring groups' satisfaction and developing actions that continually improve services. Groups served include employees, managers, executives, vendors, and physicians. Indirect groups served include patients, Board members, and others.

6. Relationships with managers, peers, etc.

This position is responsible for developing and maintaining open, honest, and mutually beneficial relationships with his or her manager, fellow managers, staff, and the departments to which he/she provides service. Relationships will be maintained in a manner consistent with Summa's mission, values, and philosophies.

7. Supporting diversity

The incumbent is responsible for ensuring a work environment within his or her department that promotes and embraces diversity.

8. Development of self and others

The incumbent is responsible for continued self-development through attendance at various Summa-sponsored management development programs, professional seminars, and conferences. Also, the incumbent is responsible for ensuring the continued development of staff.

9. Communication

The incumbent is responsible for ensuring excellent open communications within the department. This includes regular staff meetings, preparation and distribution of minutes, and other means to keep the department informed on a timely basis. The incumbent will communicate effectively with his or her manager, other members of Summa Management Team, employees, and outside customers.

10. Regulatory compliance

The incumbent is responsible for complying with regulatory and accreditation requirements through completion of Summa's mandatory organizational education, JCAHO, Code of Conduct, and compliance training. Incumbent is also responsible for adherence to Summa's mandatory organizational education requirements, JCAHO standards, Code of Conduct, and Compliance Plan in daily activities and work processes.

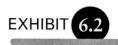

EXHIBIT 6.2 **Sample position description for director of nursing education and staff development (cont.)**

Specific key result and accountability areas essential for position

Insert the 5 or 6 key result and accountability areas in this section. These should be the major categories of responsibility for this position. Under each heading, summarize in 3–4 sentences the accountability and expectation.

1.   Education programs/services for Department of Patient Care Services
The incumbent facilitates orientations, curriculums, inservices, professional community workshops, mandatory BLS/ACLS/NPR/NVCI programs, and competency system for direct patient care providers. Teaches in selected programs.

2.   Continuing education
The incumbent oversees continuing nursing education (CE) application system for selected educational programs following the Ohio Nurses Association's CE Providership Guidelines.

3.   Policy and procedure writing
The incumbent oversees the writing and revising of the Department of Patient Care Services policies and procedures.

4.   BLS/ACLS/Crisis intervention, neonatal resuscitation, and fetal monitoring
The incumbent oversees mandatory BLS/ACLS/Crisis intervention, neonatal resuscitation, and fetal monitoring courses. The incumbent teaches BLS.

5.   Patient education
The incumbent ensures a system that assists clinical nursing personnel to develop/purchase materials to teach patients/populations of patients.

6.   Affiliating clinical rotations
The incumbent collaborates with the community Colleges/Universities of Nursing and Medical Assistant programs to provide Educational Clinical Experiences/Activities of mutual concern/need.

7.   Clerical support to achieve strategic hospital goals/education program
The incumbent supports strategic hospital goals by providing clerical support to all departments, by the running of compliance statistics for Mandatory Organizational Education and Code of Conduct, BLS/ACLS stats, employee educational records for performance appraisals, and by providing student and guest housing facilities.

Note: The above stated duties are intended to outline those functions typically performed by the incumbent in this position. This description of duties is not intended to be all-inclusive or to limit the discretionary authority of supervisors to assign additional tasks of a similar nature or level of responsibility.

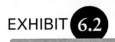

EXHIBIT **6.2** **Sample position description for director of nursing education and staff development (cont.)**

BACKGROUND, EXPERIENCE, AND EDUCATION

1. **Experience**
   Five (5) years related professional experience, including two (2) years in a supervisory or management capacity.

2. **Education and training**
   Master's degree in Nursing or related field.
   Registered Nurse with Baccalaureate degree in Nursing.

3. **Skills/Competencies**
   - Ability to direct the work effort of others through teamwork and building.
   - Ability to communicate verbally and in writing with physicians, hospital staff, educational institution representatives, and professional group representatives.
   - Ability to assess, implement, and evaluate educational needs and programs designed to meet needs of staff, patients, families, physicians, and nursing and allied health students.
   - Ability to work collaboratively with nursing personnel, physicians, hospital departments, and community institutions' representatives.

4. **Population specific competency (change wording as necessary)**
   The incumbent will have the ability to effectively interact with populations of patients/customers, with the understanding of their needs for self-respect and dignity.

5. **Other qualifications**
   - Ability to use computer and audiovisual equipment.
   - Ability to manage multiple projects at one time.

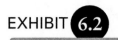

EXHIBIT **6.2** **Sample position description for director of nursing education and staff development (cont.)**

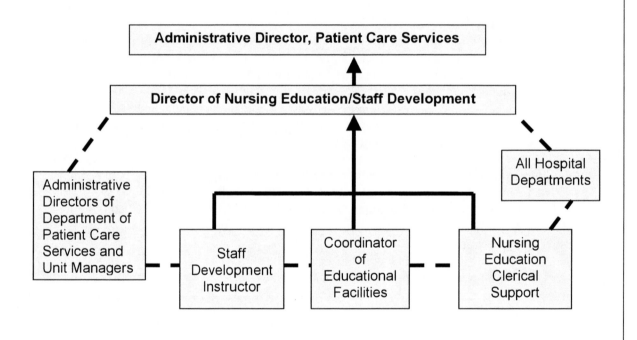

SUMMA HEALTH SYSTEM ORGANIZATION CHART

The organizational chart should accurately reflect the reporting relationships within the department. It should include what position this position reports to and any direct or indirect reports to this position.

Administrative Director, Patient Care Services

Director of Nursing Education/Staff Development

Administrative Directors of Department of Patient Care Services and Unit Managers

Staff Development Instructor

Coordinator of Educational Facilities

Nursing Education Clerical Support

All Hospital Departments

© 2005. Summa Health System. Reproduced with permission

References

Brunt, B. A. 1998. "Structure and process: New models of nursing and clinical staff development." In K. J. Kelly-Thomas. *Clinical and Nursing Staff Development: Current Competence, Future Focus.* 2nd ed. pp. 25–53. Philadelphia: Lippincott, Williams & Wilkins.

Summa Health System. 2000. Position description for Staff Development Instructor. Akron, OH: Author.

Summa Health System. 2005. Position description for Director of Nursing Education and Staff Development. Akron, OH: Author.

Orientations for
new educators

Orientations for
new educators

Learning objective

After reading this chapter, the participant should be able to
- create an orientation plan for a new educator

Using the checklist to create an orientation

Orientation programs are designed to familiarize and socialize new educators to the environment and culture in which they will practice. Planned, structured orientation programs are essential for staff new to the facility or new to the education department.

> **TIP** When designing an orientation program:
> - Provide the educator with a copy of the position description
> - Review specific considerations for all populations with whom the employee will be expected to interact on a regular basis
> - Review departmental and organizational policies and procedures
> - Include information on data management and recordkeeping

- Review any specific regulatory requirements
- Include information on the performance improvement process
- Schedule time to meet with key stakeholders
- Allow sufficient time to assimilate new information and develop necessary skills

Administrators or institutions can use the competencies tool to plan an orientation program for a new educator. Specific job expectations and competencies can be identified, and the performance criteria can be used to plan experiences to meet those expectations. Since the competencies are categorized by the roles identified in the ANA standards for NPD (2000), experiences relating to various aspects of the educational role can be included.

With individuals new to an educational role, the emphasis should be on the educator competencies rather than the other roles, but the orientation can be tailored to meet the needs of the individual educator. If the individual educator completes the tool as a self-assessment prior to the orientation, the orientation can be planned to ensure the educator gains experience in areas of identified needs.

Figure 7.1 shows how an orientation program could be established using these competencies. Another format that could be used for an orientation program is provided in Exhibit 7.1.

FIGURE **7.1**

Example of an orientation program based on selected competencies

Category and competency	Resources/experiences to meet competency
Educator: Designs and revises education activities; identifies of individual unit needs	- Review materials on adult learning principles - Read Chapters 10 and 12 in Core Curriculum - Observe planning and implementation of educational program - View videotape on teaching adults
Educator: Uses a variety of teaching strategies and audiovisuals	- Spend time with media expert or experienced educator to learn about AV equipment/resources - Read Chapter 11 in Core Curriculum - Review AV design information
Educator: Conducts needs assessment using a variety of strategies	- Read Chapter 9 in Core Curriculum - Review completed needs assessments, results, and communication strategies - Complete needs assessment for one area of responsibility
Researcher: Supports integration of research into practice	- Review evidence-based practice information - Incorporate current research data into presentations and own practice - Encourage critical thinking - Develop information to assist staff evaluation of research articles
Facilitator: Identifies internal and external resources available for staff	- Spend time with another educator to identify internal resources - Identify resources on the Internet - Gather information about professional organizations with an educational component or focus - Meet with key stakeholders/individuals to better understand their roles in the organization
Consultant: Participates in committees, task forces, projects, etc.	- Observe various committee meetings - Work with colleagues on a group project - Watch video on conducting effective meetings - Develop agenda for a meeting

FIGURE 7.1 **Example of an orientation program based on selected competencies (cont.)**

Category and competency	Resources/experiences to meet competency
Leader: Maintains required documentation and recordkeeping system	- Review Chapter 20 in Core Curriculum - Read recordkeeping policies and procedures for department - Review continuing education files/reports - Complete file for program taught
Doing the right thing: Maintains confidentiality and integrates ethical principles in all aspects of practice	- Review organizational policies and procedures on confidential information - Review Chapter 5 in Core Curriculum - Do not include identifying information on class materials or in presentation
Doing the right thing: Promotes a safe and healthy work environment	- Review appropriate safety regulations, e.g., OSHA, JCAHO - Identify unsafe work practices - Role model healthy behaviors and lifestyle
Right person doing it: Maintains educational or clinical competencies appropriate for role	- Identify required competencies - Maintain skills required for role - Develop plan to achieve competencies

EXHIBIT 7.1   **Sample orientation schedule for new OB instructor**

Summa Health System Hospitals
Nursing Education and Staff Development
Orientation for OB Instructor

Week 1

Monday, August 7, 2006

7:30–8:00 a.m.	Welcome—get keys and settle into office	Room 227
8:00–11:00 a.m.	Educational Leadership Meeting	CR C
11:00 a.m.–12:00 p.m.	Lunch with all the Staff Development Instructors	

12:00–1:00 p.m.	Meet with Staff Development Instructor regarding:
	    Nursing Assistant Orientation
	    Unit Secretary Orientation
	    Behavioral Health Workshop
		Room 228

1:00–2:00 p.m.	Meet with Senior Administrative Secretary regarding:
	    Supplies Typing requests
	    Time requests Voice mail
	    E-mail Registration process
		SD Office

2:00–4:00 p.m.	Attend DOVE update for WH Services	Bsmt Aud

Tuesday, August 8, 2006

7:00–7:30 a.m.	Meet with Night Shift Staff Development Instructor Night Shift Staff Development Instructor role	Room 233
7:30–8:00 a.m.	Go through e-mails	Room 227

8:00–9:00 a.m.	Meet with Patient Education Coordinator regarding:
	    Patient education
	    Ambulatory workshop
		Room 230

9:00–10:00 a.m.	Meet with Educational Facilities Coordinator regarding:
	    Room/AV requests
	    Building issues
		Room 104

EXHIBIT 7.1   Sample orientation schedule for new OB instructor (cont.)

10:00–11:00 a.m.	Meet with Director regarding:
	    Mission, philosophy, objectives of department
	    Organization
	    Overview of programs
		Room 101

11:00 a.m.– 12:00 p.m.	Lunch	

12:00 – 1:00 p.m.	Meet with Director regarding:
	    Resources—Phone list
	    Clinical descriptions
	    Monthly calendar
	    Staff Development Core Curriculum
		Room 101

1:00–2:00 p.m.	Meet with Staff Development Instructor regarding:
	    ACLS
	    BLS
		Room 102

2:00–3:00 p.m.	Meet with Staff Development Instructor regarding:
	    Critical Care course
	    Joe Harp conference
	    Peripheral Vascular workshop
		Room 232

3:00–3:30 p.m.	Catch up	

Thursday August 10, 2006

7:00–7:30 a.m.	Meet with Night Shift Staff Development Instructor Night Shift Staff Development Instructor role	Room 237
7:30–8:00 a.m.	Review e-mail, voice mail, etc.	Room 227
8:00–9:00 a.m.	Meeting with Clinical Director for Women's Health Expectations of Staff Development Instructor	Nursing Admin

9:00–10:00 a.m.	Meet with Director regarding:
	    Policy/procedure system
	    Clinical rotation schedule
	    Preceptor workshop
	    Nursing student tech orientation
		Room 101

EXHIBIT 7.1 **Sample orientation schedule for new OB instructor (cont.)**

10:00–11:00 a.m.	Meet with Director regarding Continuing Education system/forms	Room 101
11:00 a.m.– 12:00 p.m.	Lunch	
12:00–1:00 p.m.	Teleseminar on promoting evidence-based practice	Room 101
1:00–2:00 p.m.	Meet with Unit Manager, Women's Surgery Unit Expectations of Staff Development Instructor	2 East office
2:00–3:30 p.m.	Review information received to date Core Curriculum	

Week 2

Tuesday, August 15, 2006

7:00–10:00 a.m.	Neonatal Resuscitation Provider Renewal Session (Observe 1 or 2 going through the renewal)	3 N Nursery
10:00 a.m.– 12:00 p.m.	Meet with previous OB Instructor Women's Health Programs	Room 227
12:00–1:00 p.m.	Lunch	
1:00–2:00 p.m.	Review e-mail, voice mail, etc.	Room 227
2:00–3:00 p.m.	Meet with Corporate Communications Staff Media Services, AV Equipment, Posters	Media–PCS Ground
3:00–3:30 p.m.	Catch up	

Thursday August 17, 2006

7:00–8:00 a.m.	Review e-mails, voicemails, etc.	Room 227
8:00–9:00 a.m.	Meet with Unit Manager Postpartum Units Expectations of Staff Development Instructor	3 North office

EXHIBIT **7.1** Sample orientation schedule for new OB instructor (cont.)

9:00–10:00 a.m.	Meet with Unit Manager Labor & Delivery and Perinatal Expectations of Staff Development Instructor	L & D office
10:00–11:00 a.m.	Meet with Medical Librarian Orientation to Medical Library	Medical Library
11:00 a.m.–12:00 p.m.	Lunch	
12:00–1:00 p.m.	Meet with Unit Manager – Special Care Nursery Expectations of Staff Development Instructor	SCN office
1:00–3:30 p.m.	Review Departmental AV Resources	Room 227

Friday August 18, 2006

7:00–9:00 a.m.	Review e-mails, voice mails, etc.	Room 227
9:00–10:00 a.m.	Meet with Staff Development Instructor regarding: RN/LPN Orientation LPN IV Therapy Course Medical/Surgical Workshops	Room 231
10:00 a.m.–3:30 p.m.	Independent study based on identified needs	

Week 3

Monday August 21, 2006

7:00–9:00 a.m.	Catch up — e-mails, voice mails, etc.	Room 227
9:00–11:00 a.m.	Meet with Jenn Doyle re: Women's Health Program	Room 227
12:00–1:00 p.m.	Meet with Director re: orientation to date	Room 101
1:00–3:30 p.m.	Review *Core Curriculum*	

EXHIBIT **7.1** **Sample orientation schedule for new OB instructor (cont.)**

Wednesday August 23, 2006

7:00–8:00 a.m.	Go through e-mails/voice mails	Room 227
8:00–11:00 a.m.	Basic Life Support HCP Renewal with new standards	CR 2/3
11:00 a.m.–12:00 p.m.	Lunch	
12:00–3:30 p.m.	Independent Study	

Thursday August 24, 2006

7:00–3:30 p.m.	Additional experiences as desired

Other experiences to be scheduled:

OB Operations – 2nd Monday of each month, 12:00–1:30 pm

September 18th – Educational Leadership

Oct. 3rd - Women's Health Seminar

October 10th and 11th – Sit through AWHONN FHM PP Course

October 13th and 21st – BLS Instructor Course

October 16th – Educational Leadership

November 2 – RN Preceptor Workshop

November – NRP Instructor Course – Children's Hospital

November – AWHONN EFM Instructor Certification - Cincinnati

References

Avillion, A. E. (Ed.). 2001. *Core Curriculum for Staff Development*. 2nd ed. Pensacola, FL: National Nursing Staff Development Organization.

Brunt, B. A. 2005. "Identifying performance criteria for staff development competencies." Unpublished master's dissertation. University of Dundee, Scotland.

Performance appraisals and professional development plans

Learning objective

After reading this chapter, the participant should be able to
- create a development plan based on performance appraisal feedback

Types of performance appraisals

Performance appraisals serve both an administrative and developmental purpose. On the administrative side, they are used for making promotion, salary, or possibly layoff decisions. For developmental purposes, the assessment can be used to identify educational needs, career planning, and leadership potential.

Performance appraisal can occur in a variety of ways:
- **Peer review:** Peer review occurs when nurses judge their peer's performance against the standards determined to constitute quality practice.

- **Management by objectives:** A results-oriented evaluation that measures employee performance relative to goals achieved or objectives attained.

- **Criterion-based evaluations:** An evaluation that measures or assesses the educator's performance in relation to well-defined requirements of the job.

- **Self-evaluation:** Educators may be asked to engage in self-evaluation as part of the performance-appraisal process. The educator and manager then compare notes and negotiate a mutually acceptable final appraisal.

TIP | Improving performance appraisals:
- Performance appraisal should be an ongoing process rather than an event
- There should be no surprises during the formal performance appraisal
- Data from competence assessment activities should be included in summary comments made on annual reviews

---

Performance appraisals for staff educators

Performance appraisal is one of the ANA's standards of professional performance for nursing professional development. NPD educators should evaluate their own nursing practice in relation to professional practice standards, relevant statutes and regulations, and maintenance of continuing professional nursing competence. Measurement criteria for this standard includes engaging in a performance appraisal on a regular basis, identifying areas of strength as well as areas in which further professional development would be beneficial. Seeking constructive feedback regarding one's own practice, taking action to achieve goals identified during the performance appraisal, and participating in peer review as appropriate are also measurement criteria.

Educators can use the performance criteria in the competency tool as documentation that they have achieved expected competencies for yearly performance appraisals. Administrators can use the criteria when evaluating performance of their staff members. Typically performance appraisals are based on the competencies included in the position description, and if the position description uses the competencies in this tool, then the performance appraisal can easily flow from this description.

Since the criteria are all measurable, the tool provides an objective assessment of staff competence. Both administrators and educators can use the tool to identify goals for professional growth for the next appraisal period.

Some organizations require documentation of achievement of selected competencies as part of the performance appraisal process. The expectations vary based on roles and responsibilities, and a sample of a competency checklist developed specifically from this tool is provided in Exhibit 8.1. Another example of an equipment-related competency is provided in Exhibit 8.2.

EXHIBIT **8.1** **Sample competency checklist**

SUMMA HEALTH SYSTEM HOSPITALS
DEPARTMENT OF EDUCATION
Designs and Revises Educational Activities
Competency Checklist

Name: _____ Title: _____ Unit: _____

CRITICAL ELEMENTS	MET	NOT MET	COMMENTS
1. Plans educational activities based on assessment data			
2. Develops objectives that are relevant, realistic, and measurable			
3. Incorporates teaching/learning strategies to address identified needs and goals			
4. Identifies quality faculty for educational activities			
5. Uses up-to-date and accurate resourses/materials in presentation			
6. Revises activities based on evaluation data			
7. Ensures required paperwork is completed to comply with agency or other regulatory requirements			

☐ **Passed**   ☐ **Needs to repeat**

Validated by: _____ Date: _____
                    (Name and title)

Developed by Staff Development 6/06
Reviewed:

Source: Summa Health System. Reprinted with permission.

EXHIBIT **8.2** **Sample equipment-related competency**

SUMMA HEALTH SYSTEM HOSPITALS
DEPARTMENT OF EDUCATION
USE OF AED FOR BLS INSTRUCTOR
Competency Checklist

Name: _____ Title: _____

Unit: _____

CRITICAL ELEMENTS	MET	NOT MET	COMMENTS
1. Reviews steps of AED algorithm: a. Assesses patient and establishes unresponsiveness			
b. Calls for EMS/defibrillator			
c. Starts CPR			
2. Turns AED on			
3. Attaches AED with pads a. Below right clavicle to right of sternum			
b. Left mid-axillary line at level of 5th intercostal space			
4. Initiates analysis			
5. Delivers shock as appropriate			
6. Reassesses or reanalyzes to potential three shocks			
7. Continues CPR for one full minute			
8. Reassesses with AED, etc.			

☐ **Passed**   ☐ **Needs to repeat**

Validated by: _____ Date: _____
          (Name and title)

Reviewed:

Source: Summa Health System. Reprinted with permission.

Since performance appraisal forms vary from institution to institution, a sample evaluation form is not included in this chapter. However, information from the competencies on the checklist can be used as a guide in determining whether individuals met the competencies included on the performance appraisal.

Professional development plans

Educators can also use this tool to create a professional development plan. Since the tool is a comprehensive description of the full range of novice-to-expert staff development practices, it is not anticipated that many educators will meet all the competencies. Individual educators can use this tool to identify areas for growth, and the performance criteria can provide a road map of steps that can be taken to meet a particular competency. This will provide a systematic plan for ongoing growth and development in a particular role.

For example, if an educator has never written a grant application and wants to write one, he or she can look at the performance criteria under that competency to determine how to proceed. Steps in the process include the following:

- Identifying potential sources of funding
- Seeking assistance from an experienced grant writer
- Determining a budget and associated expenses for the project
- Assisting with or completing a grant proposal according to guidelines
- Describing other funding sources/how project will continue after funding expires
- Writing or assisting with writing a report of findings to the funding agency

The development plan should include experiences needed to gain the required skills, as well as specific timelines to achieve those skills.

TIP | Including specific deadlines can help avoid procrastination.

Reflect on development

Critical reflection is an important aspect of creating a professional development plan. Educators need to contemplate and reflect on their past experiences as they develop a plan. Identify areas of strength, as well as areas that may require further development. Critically analyzing specific situations can help identify different ways of dealing with a similar situation if it occurs again.

Some of the qualities that enable reflection include:

- Having an open mind
- Being responsible
- Considering all sides of the situation
- Considering outcomes of actions
- Taking active control of one's own education, development, and practice

Using a professional development plan provides a road map for future learning opportunities and professional growth.

References

Brunt, B. A. 2005. "Identifying performance criteria for staff development competencies." Unpublished master's dissertation. University of Dundee, Scotland.

Summa Health System. 2004. Use of AED for BLS Instructor Competency Checklist. Akron, OH: Summa Health System.

Summa Health System. 2006. Designs and Revises Educational Activities Competency Checklist. Akron, OH: Summa Health System.

University of Dundee Centre for Medical Education. 1998. Nursing and Midwifery Degree Programme: Clinical Supervision. Dundee, Scotland: Author.

Professional portfolios

Learning objective

After reading this chapter, the participant should be able to

- develop a professional portfolio

Key concepts

The following definition of portfolio from the ANA standards is presented to guide the discussion in this chapter.

Portfolio: Material documenting the professional development, career planning, demonstration of learning, and maintenance of continuing professional nursing competence of the individual nurse.

Why create a portfolio?

One of the ANA standards of professional performance for nursing professional development is that the NPD educator acquires and maintains current knowledge and competency in NPD practice. One of the measurement criteria for this standard is to maintain a personal portfolio that documents ongoing, continuing professional nursing competence. Educators need to develop their portfolio, in addition to helping nurses and other staff members develop their own portfolios.

Although portfolios currently are not widely utilized in the United States, they will become more prevalent in the future. Since 1995, the United Kingdom Central Council for Nursing, Midwifery and Health Visiting (UKCC) has required individuals on the professional register to use a Personal Professional Profile. A personal portfolio is a private collection of evidence that demonstrates the continuing acquisition of skills, knowledge, attitudes, understanding, and achievement. It is both retrospective and prospective, as well as reflecting the current stage of development of the individual. Portfolios enable individuals to keep a record of their personal and professional development, professional experiences, and qualifications.

Portfolios may include the following components:
- Professional credentials
- Continuing education
- Leadership activities
- Narrative self-reflection of practice
- Documentation of the relevance of professional learning experiences
- Examples demonstrating competence in a certain area

Creating a profile is an excellent opportunity for individuals to take stock of their life and career in the context of their future educational and work-related activities. Although some people may have already given a great deal of thought to their future career options, many have not spent time focusing on the direction they would like to take. It is worth investing time in reviewing one's situation to ensure that choices are genuine, realistic, and achievable.

TIP | Taking the time to develop a portfolio is a great way to invest in oneself and one's career.

When making decisions about future career options, individuals need to think about the personal values and interests they need to satisfy in order to be fulfilled and happy in what they choose to do. Values affect how individuals communicate with others, and they have a strong influence on personal and professional decisions. Professional values to consider are listed in Figure 9.1.

FIGURE **9.1** **Professional values to consider**

Promotion	Money
Working conditions	Hours
Helping others	Relationships
Recognition	Learning
Security	Time
Stress-free work	Diversity
Freedom	Admiration
Manager	Practitioner
Other values that are important	

Building a portfolio

The actual construction and organization of a portfolio varies depending on the individual and the organization's requirements. A portfolio generally should include the following information:

- Introduction
- Details of professional experience, knowledge, and skills
- Demonstration of achievement of required competencies
- Testimonials, references, or samples of work

Developing a portfolio provides individuals with the opportunity to be creative and include materials unique to them. Examples could include reports, research data, educational programs designed, lesson plans, and other material, as well as photographs, articles, poems, or short stories.

TIP | When building a portfolio, keep the following in mind:

- **Be selective:** Only include relevant material
- **Be clear and concise:** Make it easy to read and understand
- **Be coherent:** Have each section flow logically from the previous section
- **Be professional:** Consider the presentation—it should be typed, grammatically correct, and have the same style throughout

---

Using a portfolio

Educators can use this tool to generate ideas about how to document achievement of a particular competency. They can also use it as a means of identifying areas for development, using strategies such as reflective practice and critical incident analysis. The professional portfolio can provide a vehicle for communicating competence, professional development, and skills that could be transferable to another area.

Helping others develop professional portfolios

In addition to developing their own personal portfolio, educators may be asked to assist others in developing portfolios. In this role, the educator will help individuals make sense of the knowledge and skills they already have, and make decisions about what should be included in the portfolio.

Helping others create portfolios involves the following skills:

- **Enabling:** Supporting individuals through the development of their portfolio. This includes active listening skills and creating an environment in which individuals are able to speak openly and in confidence about their thoughts and feelings.

- **Educational counseling:** Helping individuals discover, clarify, assess, and understand their learning in order to plan realistic educational aims and career goals.

- **Advising:** Helping individuals interpret information and make decisions based on their planned learning needs.

- **Assessing:** Assisting individuals to develop confidence in self-assessment and to evaluate the scope of their learning. Through self-assessment, individuals will be much more likely to take control of the profile, make informed choices about what it should include, and have ownership of it.

- **Informing:** Providing information about learning opportunities and professional development policies.

Questions to ask the individual developing the portfolio include the following:

1. Why are you developing a portfolio?
2. What do you know about the process of developing a portfolio?
3. When do you need/want the portfolio to be completed?
4. What type of portfolio do you want?
5. What skills do you already have to complete it?
6. What skills do you need to develop?
7. How would you like me to help you with this process?
8. What help can you expect from others?

Establish an action plan with timelines and ground rules to ensure completion of the portfolio within the desired time frame.

References

American Nurses Association. 2000. *Scope and Standards of Practice for Nursing Professional Development*. Washington, DC: ANA.

Hull, C., and Redfern, L. 1996. *Profiles and Portfolios: A Guide for Nurses and Midwives*. London: Macmillan Press.

Documenting cultural competence

Learning objective

After reading this chapter, the participant should be able to

- discuss the importance of cultural competence in the educational role

Key concepts

The following definitions of key concepts are presented to guide the discussion:

Culturally competent care: Care that adapts interventions to the cultural needs and preferences (ethnic and religious beliefs, values, and practices) of a diverse group of patients.

Cultural competence: An ongoing process in which the healthcare provider continuously strives to effectively work within the cultural context of the client. This includes the integration of cultural awareness, cultural desire, cultural knowledge, cultural skills, and cultural encounters.

Cultural competence and NPD educators

Cultural competence builds first on an awareness of one's own cultural perspective, and then adds knowledge about the perspective of another culture on the same issue. Next, the person acquires the skills he or she needs when working and communicating with a member of another culture. Sharing, respecting, and integrating perspectives is important to working effectively with a diverse group of persons and developing cultural competence. Since NPD educators teach learners who represent a variety of cultures, they need to consider the effect culture has on learning.

The first plank of the ANA Code of Ethics states that the nurse, in all professional relationships, practices with compassion and respect for the inherent dignity, worth, and uniqueness of every individual, unrestricted by considerations of social or economic status, personal attributes, or the nature of health problems. One of the measurement criteria for the ANA standard on identification of educational outcomes is that educational objectives are culturally appropriate.

The first step to ensuring cultural competence is a cultural assessment, which includes the following:

- Identification of the learner's cultural understanding and norms
- Identification of learner beliefs, values, and practices that could assist or interfere with learning
- Awareness of the educator to better understand the learner's frame of reference

Too often health professionals form their own cultural perspectives, fail to modify their approaches to be responsive to the needs of culturally diverse learners, and fail to recognize the ineffectiveness of their teaching. Many nurses identify a lack of knowledge, skills, and confidence to care for patients from diverse backgrounds, and cultural content in many nursing school curriculums is limited.

Studies have demonstrated the positive impact of training in improving the cultural competence of healthcare providers. Training has been shown to improve communication across cultural and linguistic differences, as well as to increase knowledge and self-efficacy.

Components of cultural competence

Components of cultural competence include cultural awareness, cultural sensitivity, cultural knowledge, cultural skills, cultural encounters, and cultural desire.

- **Cultural awareness** requires the examination of personally held beliefs about other cultures, as well as the development of an appreciation for the values, beliefs, and life practices of those cultures.

- **Cultural sensitivity** is the awareness by an individual of his or her culture and the cultural values and beliefs of another and how these intersect. This includes openness, appreciation of another's perspective, holistic communication, genuine interest, and being nonjudgmental about others.

- **Cultural knowledge** is an active process of obtaining an educational foundation about specific physical, biological, and physiological differences.

- **Cultural skill** is the process of gathering relevant cultural data and performing cultural assessments.

- **Cultural encounters** are interactions between two or more individuals from different cultural backgrounds.

- **Cultural desire** is the willingness and motivation of the individual to participate in the process of cultural competence.

Barriers to cultural competence

- Lack of awareness of differences
- Lack of time
- Ethnocentrism, bias, and prejudice
- Lack of skills to address differences
- Lack of organizational support

Strategies to promote cultural competence

NPD educators can play a key role in improving cultural competence. Suggested topics to include in education are the relevance of cultural competence, culture and health culture, intercultural communication, language issues, and skills application.

Lack of cultural awareness of both educators and staff can be overcome with information and resources about different cultures, including using speakers from various ethnic and cultural groups. Educators may encounter resistance and be told that there is no time for such programs, but this can be overcome by changing the healthcare providers' mindset and encouraging them to put themselves in their patients' shoes, thereby allowing them to identify potential needs.

Ethnocentrism is the belief in the superiority of one's own ethnic group, which can lead to bias and prejudice against individuals who are not of the same ethnic group. Focusing on intercultural communication skills can help combat this problem, as can teaching skills to address differences, which can be part of the overall cultural awareness campaign.

Many staff members are not aware of the cultural diversity resources available. Most organizations have a number of resources available on cultural competence, including policies and procedures, resource materials, individuals with expertise in that area, and language-interpreting services.

NPD educators can document cultural competence by preparing and presenting information for staff on this topic, or by describing a situation where they addressed cultural competence in an educational program.

References

American Nurses Association. 2001. *Code of Ethics for Nurses with Interpretive Statements.* Washington, DC: American Nurses Association.

American Nurses Association. 2000. *Scope and Standards of Practice for Nursing Professional Development.* Washington, DC: American Nurses Association.

Avillion, A. E. 2004. *A Practical Guide to Staff Development: Tools and Techniques for Effective Education.* Marblehead, MA: HCPro.

Gray, D. P. 2006. "Critical reflections on culture in nursing." *Journal of Cultural Diversity* 13 (2), 76–82.

Narayan, M. C. 2003. "Cultural assessment and care planning." *Home Healthcare Nurse* 21 (9): 611–618.

Taylor, R. 2005. "Assessing barriers to cultural competence." *Journal for Nurses in Staff Development* 21 (4): 135–142.

SECTION III

Future trends

This section discusses other uses for these competencies and future trends in the field of Nursing Professional Development.

■

Potential applications of the competencies

By Julia Aucoin, DNS, RN-BC, CNE

Learning objective

After reading this chapter, the participant should be able to
- identify at least three applications of the competencies

This chapter focuses on other ways the competencies may be used. Some of the suggested applications are logical and some are provocative, to spur the consideration of new and creative uses. Each section also will describe what is needed to make the application work.

Graduate nursing education programs

Recently there has been a resurgence of graduate nursing education programs focusing on both the academic nurse educator and the staff development roles. Content for these programs should be evidence-based, as are these competencies, and consequently these competencies can be incorporated in graduate education programs. The competencies can be used in a balanced approach, and the role of the academic educator can be compared and contrasted to that of the staff development educator.

Educators can create exercises in which learners self-assess, discuss the applicability of each competency, create a competency checklist to use in the graduate practicum, or write a development plan for all or a portion of the listed competencies. This will allow the competencies to be developed, embraced, and employed when students enter the practice setting. The graduate course in staff development can be organized around the competencies to be sure that essential content is covered and course objectives are reasonable. It is necessary then that the graduate nursing education program recognize the validity of both the academic and practice roles and present them with similar evidence.

Scope and Standards of Nursing Professional Development

The American Nurses Association's *Scope and Standards of Practice for Nursing Professional Development* was last published in 2000. The competencies should be used to revise this document so that it examines the current six roles of the nursing professional development specialist (educator, leader, facilitator, change agent, researcher, and consultant), and so that the competencies are reflected in those roles, that they are fully described in the scope of practice, and that they are embedded in the standards.

Much of the existing *Scope and Standards* was based on the practice experience of educators who were chosen to develop the document. However, in 2005, the National League for Nursing published *The Scope of Practice for Academic Nurse Educators* and fully incorporated the developed competencies into the document (NLN 2005). Therefore, the revision of the *Scope and Standards* should incorporate these competencies as part of the essential content. This requires the content expert panel to have knowledge of these competencies and to acknowledge their contribution.

Resource for certification exam

These competencies should be used as a resource for the nursing professional development certification exam prepared by the American Nurses Credentialing Center. The content expert panel should include them as a reference for item development and study materials.

In addition, the test plan should be examined to be sure that it reflects the competencies. The next time a practice analysis is undertaken by the panel, the competencies can be used as a source on which to base the role analysis functions.

At a minimum, the competencies should be included as part of certification preparation courses. These courses often enroll both candidates who plan to take the certification test and those who are simply new to the role and would like an orientation to the job functions.

To accomplish the synergy with the certification exam, the members of the content expert panel team need to acknowledge that competencies are a major part of demonstrating the role of the nursing professional development specialist and adopt them as a part of the literature supporting the role.

Job function analysis

As society becomes more complex and job functions become more specialized, positions are reevaluated for appropriate title, responsibilities, and salary. Human resource departments can use the competencies as an evidence-based tool to help them perform this job analysis function.

Additionally, employees who work in staff development often perform above and beyond the job requirements, putting in long hours, taking on multiple assignments, and teaching at odd hours in order to fulfill all six roles of the NPD specialist. Using the competencies as a management tool to assign how much time or what percentage of the job should be spent on each of the key areas would be a helpful organizational tool. For this to occur, the staff development specialist should bring this document to the attention of human resources and managers so that they can employ an evidence-based approach to job function analysis.

Development plan for new role

A simple and logical application of the competencies is to create a development plan for new hires into the staff development department. Ideally, those hired into the department already possess qualifications that incorporate these factors; however, often an experienced clinician is transferred to the educator role without the necessary skills. The competencies can be used to guide both the job orientation and the staff member's development in the role. Unit-based educators would also benefit from using a portion of the competencies to guide their movement from a clinical role into a teaching role.

Facilities often hire academic educators to function in the practice development role, but the strategies and learning outcomes used by academic educators can be different from those of NPD educators. Using the competencies to orient the academic educator will help them make a successful transition. Agreeing to meet the competencies could be a prerequisite of accepting the job role, and then strategies based on the competencies could be employed to assist in the acquisition of these skills.

ANCC Magnet Recognition Program®

The American Nurses Credentialing Center's Magnet Recognition Program® includes a Force of Magnetism known as "Nurse as Teacher." One expectation of this Force is that the organization provides evidence of broad participation in professional development programs designed to develop, refine, and enhance teaching experiences to nurses who teach patients, other nurses, and students. Excerpts from the competencies can be used as a portion of a skills or competency development plan, and can be used to develop subsequent checklists or job descriptions and performance appraisals, to document that teaching competencies have been met. Not all hospitals seek ANCC Magnet Recognition®, but many use the Forces of Magnetism to guide their professional practice environment. This requires acknowledgement that the competencies are a guide for all nurses for selected teaching functions.

Need for additional research

Although the development and suggested applications of the competencies were based on multiple research studies, the work has only just begun. Further inquiry into the role of staff development, how the practice changes over time, the importance of one function over another, and comparison to academic and patient educator roles should be conducted.

The practice of staff development should be built on evidence-based teaching, and we must start with further examination of these competencies. Therefore, funded studies that look at the evidence behind practice-teaching competencies will support further development of these competencies. This requires an acknowledgement that practice education is a specialty unto itself, that good clinicians can become good teachers with specialized training, and that teaching in a practice setting requires more psychomotor and affective interactions than cognitive activities.

These applications are not exhaustive, but they promote concrete applications for the competencies. In order for research to be useful, users must have a vision of what can happen as a result of further study. Teaching in a practice setting now has a solid evidence base for job descriptions, standards, performance evaluations, development plans, and further development of standards and certification. It is the intent of this section to stimulate the reader to think of other good applications for this work.

References

American Nurses Association. 2000. *Scope and Standards of Practice for Nursing Professional Development*. Washington, DC: American Nurses Association.

American Nurses Credentialing Center. 2004. *Magnet Recognition Program*®. Washington, DC: American Nurses Association.

National League for Nursing. 2005. *The Scope of Practice for Academic Nurse Educators*. New York: National League for Nursing.

National League for Nursing. 2005. *Core Competencies of Nurse Educators*. New York: National League for Nursing. Retrieved November 15, 2006, from *www.nln.org/profdev/ corecompetencies.pdf*.

APPENDIX

Nursing professional development competency tool

Nursing Professional Development Educator Competencies

Personal Assessment of Competency

Directions: Place a check mark in the column to indicate competencies you have achieved.

Performance criteria are included with each competency statement, and you can use these as a guide to determine whether you have met a specific competency. The competencies included, which represent all levels of practice from novice to expert (Benner 1984), have been classified by Harden's (1999) outcome model and the roles identified in the ANA (2000) standards for nursing professional development.

The competencies listed will not be applicable in every setting, and can be tailored to meet the individual's needs.

List of competencies (comp) and performance criteria statements	✔ if comp met
"Doing the Right Thing" Competencies - Educator Role	

1. Designs and revises educational activities
 	
   a. Plans education activities based on assessment data
   b. Develops objective that are relevant, realistic, and measurable
   c. Incorporates teaching/learning strategies to address identified needs and goals
   d. Identifies qualified faculty for educational activities
   e. Uses up-to-date and accurate resources/materials in presentation
   f. Revises activities based on evaluation data
   g. Ensures required paperwork is completed to comply with agency or other regulatory requirements	

2. Uses a variety of teaching strategies and audiovisuals
 	
   a. Bases audiovisuals on the size of the group, setting, and equipment available
   b. Selects teaching methodology on desired learning outcome(s), learner needs, and environmental constraints	

c. Ensures audiovisuals are easily read, attractively designed, and have current content d. Uses a variety of teaching strategies to get learners actively involved e. Ensures audiovisual equipment is operational, troubleshooting as necessary f. Promotes critical thinking, application, and synthesis of knowledge g. Evaluates the effectiveness of teaching strategies during and after the presentation	✔ if comp met
3. Uses and evaluates material resources and facilities a. Plans activities based on available resources (money, equipment, etc.) b. Ensures adequate space is available for planned number of people and activities c. Seeks ways to help defray costs if appropriate (vendors, etc.) d. Gives participant opportunity to provide feedback on facilities and teaching methods e. Provides input or prepares budget and/or cost-benefit analysis	
4. Conducts needs assessments using a variety of strategies a. Identifies target audience before conducting needs assessment b. Collects assessment data from participants and other sources at regular intervals c. Uses a variety of data collection methods, based on resources and constraints, to identify needs d. Validates needs assessment data with administration and target group e. Incorporates needs assessment data into educational plan	
5. Involves learners in assessment of needs and identification of outcomes a. Collects data from members of the target audience b. Asks learners to identify their own learning needs	

    Competencies for Staff Educators: Tools to Evaluate and Enhance Nursing Professional Development

	☑ if comp met
c. Uses data from a variety of sources (e.g., performance appraisal, quality improvement data, manager feedback) to validate needs d. Validates whether learning outcomes were achieved through participant feedback, follow-up activities, etc.	

6. Determines and revises priorities for scheduled and unscheduled educational activities
 	
    a. Plans educational activities based on assessment data and organizational priorities
    b. Adjusts schedule as needed to meet needs of customers
    c. Alters educational plans as necessary to address changing circumstances
    d. Considers deadlines and time constraints when organizing and prioritizing work to be done
    e. Develops programs as needed to ensure staff members comply with current regulations, e.g., JCAHO competencies, population-specific care	

7. Evaluates effectiveness and outcomes of educational endeavors
 	
    a. Collaborates with organizational leaders and stakeholders to measure program outcomes
    b. Uses qualitative and quantitative approaches to evaluate program effectiveness
    c. Completes a cost-benefit analysis of selected programs
    d. Links program outcomes to changes in performance and/or return on investment
    e. Shares evaluation data with individuals/organization
    f. Uses customer feedback to drive program improvement	

8. Coordinates complex educational offerings
 	
    a. Develops programs based on organization's strategic plan
    b. Uses systematic approach to measure program outcomes
    c. Collaborates with appropriate stakeholders and participants to improve program design	

d. Makes judgments about quality of consequences, outcomes, and effects, or merit of program e. Reports program outcomes related to changes in performance	✔ if comp met
9. Selects appropriate teaching strategies to facilitate behavioral change a. Identifies potential barriers to successful application of knowledge b. Develops programs that address participants' beliefs and attitudes c. Allows time for behavior change or application of knowledge to take place d. Reinforces information as needed to change behavioral practice e. Documents effectiveness of programs designed to produce behavioral change	
10. Develops curriculums (classes or courses around a common theme) a. Develops program to meet organizational goals and objectives b. Identifies needs of target audience and organization c. Develops a conceptual framework for the curriculum d. Incorporates curricular threads (e.g., care across the lifespan, critical thinking, customer service) e. Plans instructional timing and sequence f. Considers process and resource management (flexible learning options, use of technology, etc.)	
11. Adjusts content and teaching strategies during presentation based on learner's reaction a. Picks up on verbal and nonverbal learner cues during sessions b. Engages the learner in educational activities c. Uses questions or other means to assess knowledge d. Alters planned strategies, if needed, based on learner response	

	☑ if comp met

12. Creates and applies newer educational methodologies
 	
    a. Uses a variety of teaching strategies, incorporating right- and left-brain approaches and methods that appeal to auditory, visual, and kinesthetic learning
    b. Networks and "borrows" ideas from colleagues
    c. Reviews resources on creative teaching and accelerated learning
    d. Uses interactive approaches to learning, including computerized instruction, if appropriate
    e. Encourages critical thinking, problem solving, and reflective reasoning	

13. Uses appropriate measurement methods to assess and document competence of personnel
 	
    a. Analyzes data (quality improvement, etc.) to determine deficits in the competence of individuals or groups
    b. Works with appropriate staff to identify competencies to be assessed
    c. Identifies clear and understandable expectations/standards for competencies
    d. Assists with designing checklists or skill inventories to assess competence
    e. Determines appropriate evaluation methods to validate competence
    f. Provides appropriate feedback on competency validation to individuals/organization	

14. Possesses expert knowledge of how to teach within organizational culture
 	
    a. Adapts strategies to the level of the learner
    b. Aligns activities with the strategic plan
    c. Demonstrates knowledge of corporate culture/chain of command
    d. Uses a team approach in planning educational activities
    e. Varies teaching strategies based on the organizational culture
    f. Solicits feedback on effectiveness from key stakeholders	

	☑ if comp met

15. Measures and communicates return on investment (ROI)
 	
    a. Identifies programs appropriate for ROI analysis
    b. Collaborates with organizational leaders in planning and implementing ROI analysis
    c. Develops an evaluation plan, including projected goals/outcomes
    d. Evaluates organizational results of training
    e. Communicates ROI to organization, department/peers, and staff	

"Doing the Right Thing" Competencies - Researcher Role	

16. Supports integration of research into practice
 	
    a. Models application of research by incorporating research into clinical presentations and practice
    b. Uses continuous quality improvement process data
    c. Creates an environment that supports individuals in critical thinking and research endeavors
    d. Encourages and supports evidence-based practice
    e. Helps staff evaluate research findings
    f. Incorporates research data into development of policies and procedures, educational standards, etc.	

17. Incorporates research findings from a variety of disciplines into programs
 	
    a. Uses research findings from other disciplines, as well as from nursing journals
    b. Incorporates research data and results into educational programs
    c. Encourages or participates in multidisciplinary research endeavors
    d. Assimilates current research from various areas into own practice to enhance teaching	

18. Assesses resources needed to facilitate research
 	
    a. Demonstrates skills in accessing literature and research findings
    b. Assists staff in identification of research or quality improvement	

	✔ if comp met
problem, design and evaluation of project, and/or application to clinical practice c. Encourages and supports research utilization and evidence-based practice d. Seeks out assistance from others (e.g., more experienced researcher, librarian, etc.) when needed e. Assists staff to access, critique and utilize research findings	
19. Develops and conducts research a. Identifies a problem, question, or hypothesis to be studied b. Reviews the literature for relevant articles on topic c. Selects research design and evaluation plan d. Writes a proposal e. Analyzes data f. Shares findings with others	
"Doing the Right Thing" Competencies - Facilitator Role	
20. Involves the client in defining problems and selecting solutions a. Collects data from clients to identify problem areas b. Assists client in identification of learning needs c. Uses data from a variety of sources (e.g., performance appraisal, quality improvement, manager feedback) to identify problem areas d. Collaborates with client or other stakeholders to identify possible solutions e. Assists with evaluation of chosen solution	
21. Collaborates within and across organization a. Identifies relevant disciplines/departments needed to achieve organizational goals b. Shares resources to achieve common goals c. Coordinates activities with the disciplines/departments d. Maintains good communication with relevant healthcare personnel/departments	

e. Assumes various roles when working with individuals or teams to promote problem solving f. Provides guidance and encourages the professional growth of others	☑ if comp met

22. Facilitates the adult learning process, creating a climate conducive to learning and fostering a good relationship with learners
 	
    a. Values each person's contribution through verbal and positive behavior recognitions (e.g., smiles, eye contact)
    b. Rewards and recognizes participants' thoughts and ideas
    c. Uses learner contributions to promote discussion
    d. Models an accepting, open approach to questions and concerns
    e. Pays attention to expressed needs/concerns
    f. Uses techniques to build trust in participants	

23. Identifies internal and external resources available for staff
 	
    a. Networks within own setting to identify internal resources
    b. Reviews current journals and catalogs for information on available resources
    c. Navigates the Internet to access resources
    d. Evaluates the applicability and validity of external resources
    e. Disseminates information on available resources to individuals within organization
    f. Networks with outside organizations/groups to identify external resources	

24. Develops sponsor relationships with business and industry
 	
    a. Identifies opportunities and benefits of collaborative endeavors with businesses and industries
    b. Participates in cooperative educational programs as appropriate
    c. Clarifies roles and expectations of all parties involved in the sponsor relationship
    d. Develops verbal or written agreement with sponsor agency
    e. Utilizes service learning (reciprocal relationship between student/employee and community where both parties engage in service and learning), if appropriate	

	☑ if comp met

25. Develops links with academia and service
 	
   a. Attends joint university/service meetings, if appropriate
   b. Promotes joint research endeavors with academia and patient care services
   c. Participates in role development of students
   d. Serves as adjunct faculty at a college or university, if appropriate
   e. Works collaboratively with academia to further service priorities
   f. Assists with orientation of clinical instructors to the facility	

"Doing the Right Thing" Competencies – Consultant Role	

26. Participates in committees, task forces, projects, etc.
 	
   a. Volunteers to serve on institutional committees and task forces
   b. Develops or follows the meeting agenda
   c. Arrives on time for each meeting and adheres to established time frame
   d. Facilitates discussion to achieve proposed goals
   e. Serves as a role model and facilitator for the meeting process
   f. Communicates progress of committee/task force to appropriate individuals	

27. Networks within and outside nursing
 	
   a. Meets others informally at workshops and other events
   b. Exchanges business cards to promote communication
   c. Identifies networking's mutual gains for both parties
   d. Utilizes knowledge gained from networking
   e. Identifies best practices as a result of networking	

28. Provides technical assistance to clients
 	
   a. Guides staff in creating and preparing materials for presentations
   b. Assists others with clinical skills in specialty practice area, if applicable
   c. Willingly shares expertise with others
   d. Mentors novice educators and staff in troubleshooting AV equipment for programs	

29. Coaches and provides feedback to improve performance
 	
  a. Works with individual(s) to identify areas for improvement or potential development
  b. Provides clear feedback and positive reinforcement to individual(s) with whom he or she is working
  c. Communicates and reinforces performance expectations
  d. Provides a supportive, nonthreatening environment for feedback and learning
  e. Facilitates learning by guiding individuals to appropriate resources for their professional development
	✔ if comp met

30. Differentiates educational problems from system problems
 	
  a. Collects data to analyze current systems and learning needs
  b. Differentiates between learning needs and non-learning needs (e.g., compliance or system problems)
  c. Assists in analyzing system problems
  d. Participates in failure mode analysis or root cause analysis to identify learning deficits
  e. Collaborates with management team to define the problem and identify solutions	

31. Uses consultation skills internally and externally
 	
  a. Gives expert advice on a topic or shares information with others
  b. Lists approaches used in assisting with problem identification or diagnosis
  c. Collaborates with key stakeholders on consultation requests
  d. Works with client to develop plan and recommend actions to deal with the identified issue
  e. Effectively communicates findings verbally and in writing to the client	

 Competencies for Staff Educators: Tools to Evaluate and Enhance Nursing Professional Development

	✔ if comp met

32. Consults on performance problems
 	
    a. Assesses and analyzes areas of performance problems
    b. Works with staff and managers to develop a plan of action to assist with remediation and/or performance deficits
    c. Provides clear feedback and positive reinforcement
    d. Identifies opportunities for staff to increase skill and competence
    e. Accurately documents performance using established criteria	

33. Conducts focus groups
 	
    a. Selects group members and facilitators
    b. Develops discussion group questions
    c. Arranges for appropriate setting for focus group meetings
    d. Creates nonthreatening and nonevaluative environment where group members can express themselves openly
    e. Compiles information into an appropriate format for review	

34. Maintains required documentation and record-keeping system
 	
    a. Ensures records are in compliance with departmental, organizational, and external agency requirements
    b. Restricts access to records only to authorized individuals
    c. Maintains confidentiality of records
    d. Ensures participant and program data is easily retrievable
    d. Creates reports to document progress toward attainment of staff development and organizational goals	

35. Facilitates team-building
 	
    a. Helps set clear goals and expectations for team
    b. Creates an open, trusting environment
    c. Assesses and develops communication and other skills of team members	

d. Teaches and facilitates team members to work together to find solutions e. Shares team successes with administration and throughout organization	☑ if comp met
36. Evaluates overall program effectiveness a. Develops programs based on the organization's strategic plan b. Uses a systematic approach to measure program outcomes and improve program design c. Uses both formative and summative evaluation information to evaluate program effectiveness d. Evaluates program's success at achieving strategic directions e. Shares evaluation data with individuals/organization	
37. Develops standards for educational practice in own setting a. Applies national standards (e.g., ANA) to specific setting b. Develops educational standards for current setting consistent with organizational goals c. Creates appropriate policies/procedures to support standards d. Communicates standards within the organization	
38. Develops or provides input into annual budget a. Analyzes previous revenues and expenses to identify budgeting needs b. Forecasts future needs based on environmental factors, strategic initiatives, and departmental goals c. Prepares budget to support goals of provider unit d. Monitors budget on a regular basis	
39. Uses appropriate measurement tools and methods in quality improvement (QI) activities a. Selects appropriate indicators to monitor quality and effectiveness of programs b. Collects data related to QI initiatives from a variety of sources c. Uses measurement tools appropriate to the solution	

 Competencies for Staff Educators: Tools to Evaluate and Enhance Nursing Professional Development

d. Analyzes data related to QI activities e. Measures improvements and monitors progress	☑ if comp met

40. Applies skill in strategic planning
 	
    a. Identifies needs
    b. Develops goals
    c. Links education to the organization's strategic plan
    d. Develops strategic plan for education department
    e. Evaluates outcomes	

41. Markets the staff development and continuing education programs
 	
    a. Identifies customer needs
    b. Develops marketing plan with established goals, activities, and projected costs
    c. Considers the four Ps of marketing (product, price, place, and promotion)
    d. Advertises program using a variety of methods and ensures all necessary information is included
    e. Collects data to monitor effectives of plan	

42. Calculates risks and benefits of educational innovations
 	
    a. Identifies pros and cons (risks and benefits) of possible teaching innovations
    b. Performs cost-benefit analysis of innovative teaching strategies
    c. Describes quality and quantity of educational outcomes
    d. Plans strategies to promote innovation
    e. Analyzes organizational readiness for change	

43. Writes grant proposals or participates in grant writing process
 	
  a. Identifies potential sources for funding
  b. Seeks assistance from experienced grant-writer, as needed
  c. Projects a budget and associated expenses for project
  d. Assists with or completes grant proposal according to guidelines
  e. Describes other funding sources/how project will continue after funding expires
  f. Writes or assists with writing report of findings to funding agency
	✔ if comp met

"Doing the Right Thing" Competencies – Change Agent Role	

44. Facilitates change
 	
  a. Works with organizational leaders and others to identify areas of needed change
  b. Serves as a positive role model for change
  c. Promotes problem solving by clarifying issues related to change process
  d. Creates an environment to support staff
  e. Works with others (administration, other disciplines, etc.) to facilitate change
  f. Evaluates the impact of change	

45. Serves as a change agent
 	
  a. Introduces and supports new ideas
  b. Facilitates research-based practice
  c. Works with others to identify problems and solutions
  d. Develops goals and evaluates effectiveness of change process
  e. Develops programs to educate staff or help staff cope with change	

"Doing the Thing Right" Competencies	✔ if comp met

46. Maintains confidentiality
 	
  a. Follows organizational policies and procedures on release of confidential information
  b. Does not use any identifying information during class discussions or in written materials
  c. Adheres to legislation relating to confidentiality (e.g., HIPAA)
  d. Emphasizes the importance of confidentiality to staff
  e. Respects individual's need for confidentiality (e.g., learner, manager)	

47. Promotes a safe and healthy work environment
 	
  a. Identifies unsafe work practices
  b. Maintains safe working environment
  c. Plans educational activities to promote safety
  d. Complies with safety regulations (OSHA, JCAHO, etc.)
  e. Models healthy behaviors and lifestyle	

48. Uses principles for theories of adult learning, organizational development, system change, and quality improvement
 	
  a. Uses education process to plan activities
  b. Connects topics with organizational mission, goals, and vision
  c. Promotes active involvement of the learner
  d. Provides for a variety of teaching strategies that promote problem solving
  e. Applies principles of continuous quality improvement to measure outcomes, trends, and/or results	

49. Integrates ethical principles in all aspects of practice
 	
  a. Maintains confidentiality
  b. Models ethical behavior
  c. Incorporates ethics and ethical principles into programs
  d. Facilitates and supports ethical decision-making by others
  e. Demonstrates honesty and integrity in practice	

50. Demonstrates expertise in use of computers
 	
  a. Assists others to develop expertise in the use of computers
  b. Demonstrates proficiency in the use of various computer programs, including e-mail and clinical information systems
  c. Uses computer-based instructional methods for programs, if available
  d. Navigates the Internet effectively and efficiently for information
	✔ if comp met

51. Maintains educational standards
 	
  a. Uses specific standards (e.g., ANA) for staff development activities
  b. Seeks or maintains certification
  c. Communicates educational standards within the organization
  d. Keeps up to date by reading journals and attending conferences	

52. Communicates effectively with all levels of organization
 	
  a. Demonstrates good oral and written communication skills
  b. Uses a variety of methods to communicate, e.g., e-mail, memo, flyer
  c. Responds appropriately to communications with timely feedback
  d. Distributes information about educational programs/events throughout organization
  e. Participates in interdisciplinary programs/teams	

53. Ensures educational programs are congruent with organizational mission and goals
 	
  a. Supports organization by incorporating vision and goals into programs
  b. Prioritizes educational offerings based on organizational needs
  c. Links programs to strategic initiatives
  d. Evaluates effectiveness of programs and organizational impact	

54. Maintains flexibility when managing multiple roles and responsibilities
 	
  a. Adjusts schedule as needed to meet needs of customers
  b. Alters educational plans as needed to meet organizational goals	

	☑ if comp met
c. Adapts to changing circumstances d. Manages change positively e. Adjusts priorities/teaching techniques to meet learner needs f. Meets deadlines by organizing and prioritizing work to be done	
55. Interprets and communicates across boundaries a. Identifies territories/groups and their values b. Respects identified boundaries c. Assesses and analyzes issues of all parties d. Maintains open communication to meet mutual goals e. Collaborates with other areas for dialogue and problem solving	
56. Accesses information external to organization a. Participates in professional organizations b. Networks with others outside institution c. Gathers information from various sources, e.g., library, individuals, organizations d. Attends outside conferences/seminars e. Reads professional journals	
57. Communicates impact of new educational strategies to others a. Uses a variety of educational methodologies b. Evaluates the effectiveness of teaching strategies used c. Shares evaluative data on teaching strategies with other educators d. Publishes successful strategies in institution newsletter or national journal	
58. Demonstrates awareness of historical and emerging trends a. Reads current literature to keep abreast of emerging trends b. Relates historic events to current practice c. Integrates research and current trends in own practice d. Builds on existing body of knowledge e. Plans programs to address forecasted trends (e.g., computer-based learning)	

59. Fosters systematic analysis of issues a. Participates in strategic planning or performance improvement teams b. Models critical thinking and analysis c. Coaches managers and others in the use of systematic analysis d. Helps develop action plan for identified areas of need	✔ if comp met
60. Mentors other professionals a. Assists in orientation of new educators/staff b. Serves as a role model for others c. Shares knowledge/ideas with person being mentored d. Uses a variety of methods to help educators/others develop skills e. Provides constructive feedback to person being mentored f. Serves as a role model for career development	
61. Critically processes information and problem-solves a. Demonstrates effective problem-solving skills b. Questions assumptions, using critical thinking skills c. Researches information d. Seeks advice/resources to make decisions e. Analyzes data	
62. Produces desired outcomes relevant to organization a. Assesses work environment, management support, and available resources b. Identifies clinical and financial indicators to monitor, trend, and track outcomes c. Analyzes staff development interventions as they relate to outcomes d. Uses methodological approaches to outcome measurement e. Links performance to outcomes using return on investment or changes in performance	

	✔ if comp met

63. Develops proactive educational policies and procedures for organization
 	
    a. Ensures policies define the scope of service to guide decisions and actions
    b. Monitors current initiatives of regulatory agencies and legislation for policy/procedure implications
    c. Develops process for periodic review and evaluation of policies and procedures
    d. Establishes policies that lay the groundwork for development of indicators to measure success and validate the quality of services	

64. Functions within the political climate of the organization
 	
    a. Collaborates with formal and informal decision-makers in the organization
    b. Builds internal and external alliances to achieve goals
    c. Demonstrates excellent communication skills
    d. Serves on key multidisciplinary committees
    e. Ensures departmental goals are congruent with organization's strategic plans	

65. Publishes information that can be used by other educators
 	
    a. Shares educational strategies or processes that worked with others
    b. Writes a query letter or discusses with peers appropriateness of information to be shared
    c. Writes a synopsis or outline of information to be included
    d. Develops/maintains Web site for sharing information
    e. Presents poster or concurrent sessions at workshops or within organization	

"Right Person Doing It" Competencies	

66. Maintains educational or clinical competencies appropriate for role
 	
    a. Identifies what competencies are needed for role
    b. Regularly assesses own competence in required skills
    c. Maintains educational skills and clinical skills, if required for role	

	✔ if comp met
d. Continues to educate self on educational technologies e. Develops plan to increase educational or clinical competence	

67. Promotes concept of lifelong learning
 	
    a. Provides a variety of ways to give and receive information
    b. Serves as a role model
    c. Publicizes learning opportunities for staff
    d. Collaborates with others to foster an environment that promotes life-long learning
    e. Develops goals based on assessment of career path	

68. Establishes credibility with other professionals
 	
    a. Demonstrates expertise/competence
    b. Listens effectively, maintaining open communication
    c. Follows through on tasks
    d. Responds to others in a timely manner
    e. Maintains confidentiality	

69. Serves as a role model for education
 	
    a. Mentors individuals/groups in educational activities
    b. Actively participates in continuing education activities
    c. Demonstrates appropriate application of adult learning principles
    d. Maintains high standards of professional behavior
    e. Attains/maintains certification
    f. Keeps up to date on current healthcare/educational issues	

70. Seeks opportunities to develop the various staff development roles as defined by the ANA
 	
    a. Assesses, plans, presents, and evaluates educational programs for staff (educator role)
    b. Assists individuals to accomplish their goals and keeps system/group processes running smoothly (facilitator role)	

	✔ if comp met
c. Identifies and initiates needed change (change agent role) d. Serves as a resource and assists individuals or groups with educational issues (consultant role) e. Promotes research, research utilization, and evidence-based practice (researcher role) f. Provides and supports administrative structures to achieve departmental and organizational goals (leader role)	

71. Participates in activities external to practice setting
 	
   a. Shares expertise with individuals outside of practice setting
   b. Gives presentations to outside groups
   c. Is an active member of professional association
   d. Participates in speaker's bureau
   e. Provides consultation to external individuals/groups/agencies	

72. Sees beyond role-established boundaries
 	
   a. Networks with other colleagues and other disciplines
   b. Accepts a variety of assignments
   c. Seeks learning opportunities inside and outside of work environment
   d. Goes beyond duties in job description to achieve organizational goals
   e. Thinks "outside the box," seeks new ways of doing things, is innovative and proactive, and has a positive attitude toward change	

© 2005 Barbara Brunt	

Nursing education instructional guide

Competencies for Staff Educators: Tools to Evaluate and Enhance Nursing Professional Development

Target audience

Directors of Education

Staff Development Specialists

Chief Nursing Officers

Directors of Nursing

Nurse Managers

VPs of Nursing

Nurse Preceptors

HR Professionals

Patient educators

Statement of need

This book is appropriate for staff development or patient educators in any setting. Individuals can take the competencies in this book and immediately incorporate them in their practice. The competencies can be used in a variety of ways, such as creating an orientation for a new staff development specialist, completing a self-assessment, creating criterion-based job descriptions, or using them as part of a performance development plan. This consistent, objective, validated tool can assist NPD personnel in measuring their competence. With today's emphasis on cost-containment and accountability, it is critical that educators demonstrate their competence. (This activity is intended for individual use only.)

Educational objectives

Upon completion of this activity, participants should be able to

- discuss key components of competence and competency-based education
- describe the research process used to develop the competencies and performance criteria
- identify how the educational competencies fit with the ANA standards, Harden's outcome model, and Benner's novice-to-expert continuum
- list at least four methods to validate competence
- complete a self-assessment using the checklist
- develop an educator position description specific to the setting
- create an orientation plan for a new educator
- create a development plan based on performance appraisal feedback
- develop a professional portfolio
- discuss the importance of cultural competence in the educational role
- identify at least three applications of the competencies

Faculty

Barbara A. Brunt, MA, MN, RN,BC, is Director of Nursing Education and Staff Development for Summa Health System Hospitals in Akron, OH. She has held a variety of staff development positions, including educator, coordinator, and director, for the past 28 years. Brunt has presented on a variety of topics both locally and nationally, and has published numerous articles and chapters in books. She served as section editor for the first and second editions of *The Core Curriculum for Staff Development*, published by NNSDO, and was part of the task force that revised the *Scope and Standards of*

Practice for Nursing Professional Development, published by ANA. She is a coauthor of the *Competency Management System: Toolkit for Validation and Assessment*, published by HCPro.

Brunt holds a master's degree in community health education from Kent State University and a master's in nursing from the University of Dundee in Scotland. Her research has focused on competencies. Brunt maintains certification in nursing professional development, as well as medical-surgical nursing. She has been active in numerous professional associations and has received awards for excellence in writing, nursing research, leadership, and staff development. Brunt is serving a term as President-Elect of NNSDO through July of 2007, when she will begin a two-year term as President of that organization.

Julia Aucoin, DNS, RN-BC, CNE, is certified in Nursing Professional Development and Academic Education and has worked on the certification teams with associated competencies for both specialty practices. She has served as a professor in nursing education and as the CE Consultant for the North Carolina Nurses Association, and has held positions as Director of Education in several hospitals. Dr. Aucoin is a frequent presenter at the National Nurses Staff Development Organization (NNSDO) and National League for Nursing's Annual Conventions as well as published author on nursing education topics. She is coeditor of *Conversations in Nursing Professional Development*.

Accreditation/designation statement

HCPro is accredited as a provider of continuing nursing education by the American Nurses Credentialing Center Commission on Accreditation.

This educational activity for three nursing contact hours is provided by HCPro, Inc.

Disclosure statements

HCPro, Inc., has a conflict of interest policy that requires course faculty to disclose any real or apparent commercial financial affiliations related to the content of their presentations/materials. It is not assumed that these financial interests or affiliations will have an adverse impact on faculty presentations; they are simply noted here to fully inform the participants.

Barbara A. Brunt and Julia Aucoin have declared that they have no commercial/financial vested interest in this activity.

Instructions

In order to be eligible to receive your nursing contact hours for this activity, you are required to do the following:

1. Read the book *Competencies for Staff Educators: Tools to Evaluate and Enhance Nursing Professional Development*
2. Complete the exam
3. Complete the evaluation
4. Provide your contact information on the exam and evaluation
5. Submit exam and evaluation to HCPro, Inc.

Please provide all of the information requested above and mail or fax your completed exam, program evaluation, and contact information to

HCPro, Inc.
Attention: Continuing Education Department
200 Hoods Lane
P.O. Box 1168
Marblehead, MA 01945
Fax: 781/639-0179

NOTE:

This book and associated exam are intended for individual use only. If you would like to provide this continuing education exam to other members of your nursing staff, please contact our customer service department at 877/727-1728 to place your order. The exam fee schedule is as follows:

Exam quantity	Fee
1	$0
2–25	$15 per person
26–50	$12 per person
51–100	$8 per person
101+	$5 per person

Continuing education exam

Name: _____

Title: _____

Facility name: _____

Address: _____

Address: _____

City: _____ State: _____ Zip: _____

Phone number: _____ Fax number: _____

E-mail: _____

Nursing license number: _____

(ANCC requires a unique identifier for each learner.)

Date completed: _____

1. **Which of the following is not a characteristic of competency-based education (CBE)?**

    a. Learner sets own pace

    b. Focus is on tasks

    c. Evaluation is normative-referenced

    d. Focus is on student outcomes

2. **A person's capacity to perform his or her job function is**

    a. performance criteria

    b. competence

    c. staff development

    d. competency statement

3. **Feedback from the 10 phases of stage 2 of the research study was obtained from**

    a. academic educators

    b. National Nursing Staff Development Organization members

    c. staff development educators

    d. nurses certified in Nursing Professional Development

4. Which of the following was NOT included in the research studies leading to the competency assessment tool?

    a. Delphi study on advanced practice competencies

    b. Pilot study to test the methodology

    c. Validation of results with academic educators

    d. Administrative feedback on staff development role

5. Authoritative statements that describe a competent level of care are

    a. standards of nursing practice

    b. standards of professional performance

    c. continuing competence

    d. performance criteria

6. Which of the following categories is NOT part of Harden's outcome model?

    a. Doing the right thing

    b. Performing the right skill

    c. Doing the thing right

    d. Right person doing it

7. Which of the following is not an American Nurses Association (ANA) standard of professional performance?

    a. Quality of practice

    b. Ethics

    c. Collaboration

    d. Diagnosis

8. According to Benner's theory, an educator who is comfortable with the application of knowledge and skills and who can set priorities is considered

    a. a novice

    b. an advanced beginner

    c. competent

    d. proficient

9. A method used to validate competence that generally uses a "met" and "not met" format and evaluates a single occurrence is a

    a. post-test

    b. case study

    c. competency checklist

    d. simulation

10. Examples of methods used to differentiate levels of competence include all of the following EXCEPT

    a. case studies

    b. mind mapping

    c. competency checklists

    d. observations of daily work

11. When completing a self-assessment, the educator should NOT

    a. focus on competencies expected in his or her role

    b. provide examples of how the criteria were met

    c. seek out experiences to develop additional skills

    d. disseminate the results

12. A criterion-based position description would focus on the

    a. organization's philosophy, mission, vision, and values

    b. goals and objectives of the education department

    c. skills required to perform the job

    d. services the education department provides

13. The organizational structure where staff development activities are performed by a core team of educators reporting to a single director is considered

    a. centralized

    b. decentralized

    c. combination

    d. matrix

14. Factors to consider when designing an orientation program for a new educator include all of the following EXCEPT

   a. Departmental policies and procedures

   b. Responsibilities outlined in position description

   c. Time to meet with key stakeholders

   d. Peer evaluation of performance

15. Developmental purposes of performance appraisals include all of the following EXCEPT

   a. identifying educational needs

   b. making promotion decisions

   c. facilitating career planning

   d. identifying leadership potential

16. A tool that includes experiences needed to gain required skills and a timeline to achieve those is called

   a. a competency checklist

   b. a professional development plan

   c. management by objectives

   d. criterion-based evaluation

17. Material documenting the professional development, career planning, demonstration of learning, and maintenance of continuing professional nursing competence is known as a

   a. portfolio

   b. professional development plan

   c. self-assessment

   d. competency checklist

18. Which of the following components is generally NOT included in a portfolio?

   a. Details of professional experience, knowledge, and skills

   b. Demonstration of achievement of required competencies

   c. Copies of performance appraisals

   d. Testimonials, references, or samples of work

19. Cultural competence includes the integration of all of the following components EXCEPT

    a. cultural awareness

    b. cultural knowledge

    c. cultural ethnocentrism

    d. cultural desire

20. One of the barriers to cultural competence is

    a. ethnocentrism

    b. awareness of differences

    c. cultural skill

    d. cultural encounters

21. Methods for applying these competencies in the graduate nursing education setting include all of the following EXCEPT

    a. creating a checklist to use in graduate practicum

    b. creating a development plan

    c. revising the scope and standards of practice

    d. discussing the applicability of competencies to the current role

22. Which one of the following is NOT included as a potential future use of these competencies?

    a. Completing a job function analysis

    b. Inclusion in the Forces of Magnetism

    c. Serving as a resource for the certification exam

    d. Creating a professional portfolio

Continuing education evaluation

Name: _____

Title: _____

Facility name: _____

Address: _____

Address: _____

City: _____ State: _____ Zip: _____

Phone number: _____ Fax number: _____

E-mail: _____

Nursing license number: _____

(ANCC requires a unique identifier for each learner.)

Date completed: _____

1. **This activity met the learning objectives stated:**

    Strongly Agree   Agree   Disagree   Strongly Disagree

2. **Objectives were related to the overall purpose/goal of the activity:**

    Strongly Agree   Agree   Disagree   Strongly Disagree

3. **This activity was related to my continuing education needs:**

    Strongly Agree   Agree   Disagree   Strongly Disagree

4. **The exam for the activity was an accurate test of the knowledge gained:**

    Strongly Agree   Agree   Disagree   Strongly Disagree

5. **The activity avoided commercial bias or influence:**

    Strongly Agree   Agree   Disagree   Strongly Disagree

 Competencies for Staff Educators: Tools to Evaluate and Enhance Nursing Professional Development

6. This activity met my expectations:

    Strongly Agree   Agree   Disagree   Strongly Disagree

7. Will this activity enhance your professional practice?

    Yes   No

8. The format was an appropriate method for delivery of the content for this activity:

    Strongly Agree   Agree   Disagree   Strongly Disagree

9. If you have any comments on this activity please note them here:

10. How much time did it take for you to complete this activity?

Thank you for completing this evaluation of our continuing education activity!

Return completed form to:

HCPro, Inc. • Attention: Continuing Education Department • 200 Hoods Lane, Marblehead, MA 01945

Telephone: 877/727-1728 • Fax: 781/639-2982